D1530758

Doctoral Education in Nursing: History, Process, and Outcome

Sylvia E. Hart, PhD, RN, Editor

Pub. No. 15-2238

National League for Nursing • New York

ISBN 0-88737-420-4

Manufactured in the United States of America

Contributors

Billye J. Brown, EdD, RN
Dean
La Quinta Centennial Professor in Nursing
The University of Texas at Austin
Austin, Texas

Mary E. Conway, PhD, FAAN
Dean and Professor
School of Nursing, Medical College of Georgia
Augusta, Georgia

Sr. Mary Jean Flaherty, PhD, RN, FAAN
Associate Professor
Director of the Doctoral Program
The Catholic University of America
Washington, DC

Patricia R. Forni, PhD, RN, FAAN
Dean
College of Nursing
The University of Oklahoma
Oklahoma City, Oklahoma

Sylvia E. Hart, PhD, RN
Dean
College of Nursing
University of Tennessee
1200 Volunteer Blvd.
Knoxville, Tennessee

Elizabeth R. Lenz, PhD, RN
Associate Dean for Graduate Studies and Professor
Director of Doctoral Program
University of Maryland
School of Nursing
655 W. Lombard Street
Baltimore, Maryland

E. Jane Martin, PhD, RN
Professor and Dean
College of Nursing
The University of Akron
206 Carroll Street
Akron, Ohio

Bonnie L. Rickelman, EdD, RN
Associate Professor
Chair, Division of Acute and Chronic Illness
Graduate Advisor, Doctoral Program
The University of Texas at Austin
Austin, Texas

Contents

Contents

Foreword

Well over half of the nearly 50 doctoral programs in nursing currently in existence were established since 1980. As we near the end of the decade, this is clearly a phenomenon worth pondering. Hence the idea behind this publication.

The contributors to this text present their insights about and perspectives on doctoral education in nursing with focus and clarity. Variations in degree designations, historical perspectives, resource issues, development of programs and proposals, readiness assessment, and the nursing faculty as a community of scholars—all topics germaine to doctoral programs in nursing—are comprehensively addressed.

All of the authors for this text have been associated with doctoral programs in nursing in significant and diverse ways. They share their considerable expertise with us in ways that will be useful not only to those with responsibility for delivering quality programs but also for those who are or who will be enrolled in them.

Sylvia E. Hart
Editor

1

The Doctor of Philosophy Degree: Evolutionary and Societal Perspectives

E. Jane Martin, PhD, RN

INTRODUCTION

Doctoral education in nursing has never been a more timely topic, and exploring the type of degree program most appropriate for the field is more significant today than ever before. The number of institutions with doctoral programs virtually exploded in the last 15 years. For example, by the end of 1974, there were 8 doctoral programs in nursing: 4 PhD, 1 EdD, and 3 professional degree granting. In 1988, to date, there are 47 such programs: 35 PhD, 1 EdD, and 12 professional degree granting. Although the number of different degrees remains great, i.e., PhD, EdD, DN, ND, DNS, DNSc, DSN, the doctor of philosophy degree remains the most popular—and esteemed—choice.

In order to understand this continued valuing of the PhD, this chapter will look at the evolution of the degree as well as examine it from a societal perspective.

THE DOCTOR OF PHILOSOPHY DEGREE

European Origins

As an earned university degree, the doctorate can be traced to the medieval European cities of Bologna and Paris during the years when the trade guilds were forming. In Bologna in the 1160s, the teachers' guild took the name *Universitas* of Doctors. The title *Doctor* was derived from the Latin word *docere*, meaning to teach, and *doctorem*, meaning teacher (Oxford English Dictionary, 1971). By 1200, a subguild called University Professors of the Civil and Canon

1

Law was formed, and by 1219 the awarding of formal degrees was in place. Meanwhile in Paris, the teaching guild, which was established in the 1170s, chose the name *masters*, from the Latin word *magister*.

From the beginning, Bologna, a city where civil and canon law were studied, called its teachers doctors, whereas Paris, a center for the study of the arts, called its faculty masters. In addition, the title of professor was also used interchangeably in both universities. Graduates had the title chosen by each university conferred upon them at graduation, and were then admitted to the local guild. Thus, earning the degree meant being admitted into the faculty of the university, or guild, by the faculty and having the license or right to teach there (Spurr, 1970).

In addition, it was fairly common for faculty to be able to teach in other universities without further examination. Following the requirement of papal approval for an institution to grant degrees (implemented during the 1220s), universities became international organizations, and their graduates were internationally sanctioned to teach at any university without further testing; it became a full right. Later, a change in control from faculty to students at the University of Bologna as well as universities in other cities resulted in the titles doctor and master thereafter representing not an office (i.e., faculty position), but a degree. Subsequently, as the number of nonteaching doctors increased, the titles lost even more importance. In contrast, professor remained a title and came to signify senior rank as a teacher (Harris, Troutt, & Andrews, 1980).

From its earliest use as an unofficial title to designate a teacher, and through the period when it actually became a degree signifying completion of study and admission to a guild, the term doctor came to convey expectations for the performance of scholarly work as well as teaching. This was especially true of the faculty of arts, as compared to the faculties of theology, medicine, and law, who prepared their students for specific vocations. The faculty of arts taught the trivium (grammar, rhetoric, and dialectic) and the quadrivium (arithmetic, geometry, astronomy, and music), which constituted the major portion of university learning (Lash, 1987).

For over 600 years, graduates of the University of Bologna were given the title doctor (or professor). The use of doctor spread throughout Italy and into Germany. During the same period, masters (or professor) was the title given to graduates from the University of Paris, and later, Oxford University. Thus, until the twentieth century, the German Doctor of Philosophy was equivalent to the English Master of Arts (Spurr, 1970).

The baccalaureate degree grew from a tradition of allowing advanced students (four or five years of study completed out of the eight required) to tutor or lecture in limited areas in a masters school; they were known as *bachalari*. By the late thirteenth century, the University of Paris was awarding the *Baccalaureat* as an inferior degree signifying the end of the first period of study and the successful completion of examinations. The student (or *baceler*, meaning young man or squire) then undertook limited teaching responsibilities while engaging in advanced study. In France, the period of study for the bachelor's degree gradually decreased and the period for the master's increased until it became the first university degree (the Baccalaureat was then earned by the student completing secondary school). However, in England the opposite occurred. Greater and greater emphasis was placed on the Bachelor of Arts degree, and the Master of Arts became a formality, as at Oxford and Cambridge today (Spurr, 1970).

In Germany, the doctorate became the first earned degree and the bachelor's degree disappeared. Not only professors but teachers in the *gymnasia* and civil servants were expected to earn the PhD. University professors were researchers who taught all students the same, expecting all to become candidates for the doctorate, even though only about 25 percent of them would enter the university as faculty, the rest entering practical fields such as secondary schools, government, and industry (Harris, Troutt, & Andrews, 1980).

Development in the United States

Higher education in America was thus shaped by very different systems of education, first from England, and later from Germany. From the founding of Harvard College in 1636 to the beginning of the Civil War some 200 years later, the English system dominated education in the United States, and the baccalaureate degree was the only earned degree awarded. The BA was earned following completion of a strictly prescribed classical course of study; "the boy being expected to adjust to the curriculum, not the curriculum to the boy" (Storr, 1953, p. 2). The Master of Arts degree was awarded *in cursu* or *pro forma* to those alumni who paid fees and qualified by "staying alive and out of trouble for three years after graduating from college" (Storr, 1953, p. 1). Neither evidence of intellectual attainment nor residence as a student was required to earn the master's during this time.

Dissatisfaction with the undergraduate college system—which consisted primarily of denominational colleges with limited curricula taught by recitation—grew as American colleges compared less and less favorably with the European universities. This, in turn, resulted in the necessity for more and more Americans to study abroad in order to receive high quality education. The German university system, the envy of the intellectual world at this time, was the choice of thousands of Americans, many of whom were excited by the freedom and challenge of the German system and surprised that the curriculum did not consist of attending class daily and memorizing, but rather studying to pass examinations. Many of these new doctors returned with a desire to modify the American system to fit the German model. This modification, however, proved to be a slow process (Harris, Troutt, & Andrews, 1980).

Berelson (1960), examining the development of graduate education in the United States, identified four factors of importance which were operating in this country prior to the founding of Johns Hopkins University in 1876—the event that marked the emergence of the German model—and which slowed the process:

- Normal resistance to innovation and change by established faculties
- Tension between scholarship and professional practice as the primary objective of graduate study
- Impact of a fast but unevenly growing body of knowledge
- Conflict between influences on educational policy from inside the academic community (the universities and the disciplines) and from outside (the needs of the times)

These four factors remain amazingly applicable today.

The following 25 years leading to the turn of the century are described as the period of university revolution. Higher education in the United States changed radically, and many of the results are still operational today. Programs of graduate study began in three kinds of institutions: new colleges or universities such as Johns Hopkins, University of Chicago, and Clark; private colleges like Harvard, Yale, Columbia, and Cornell; and public institutions such as California, Michigan, and Wisconsin (Berelson, 1960). Yale awarded the first PhD in 1861.

Efforts to build an exclusively graduate university culminated in the opening of Johns Hopkins University in 1876 (Brodie, 1986). Clark and the University of Chicago also tried to develop graduate only institutions, but all three eventually succumbed to practicalities of the time and place—e.g., economics, service to the community, need to develop a supply of graduate students—and the compromise was a graduate school based on the German model being placed on an undergraduate college based on the English model. Adding graduate work as another layer led to organizational decisions that are still in operation today. For example, undergraduate and graduate faculties were intermingled which resulted in undergraduate teaching methods such as required class attendance, course examinations, grades, and lectures following the undergraduate faculty to the graduate level as they moved up in the system (Berelson, 1960).

Another lasting result of this period was the hard-fought decision to place the emphasis on new scientific knowledge rather than the traditional curriculum. In the beginning, the new scientific learning was introduced and facilitated through grant moneys to Harvard and Yale. Eventually, scientific courses and areas of study were accepted and the scientific approach permeated other subjects: e.g., social studies became social sciences and philosophy lost psychology to science and became more positivistic. Berelson points out "that the graduate school came into being under the pressure of science and that it has lived its whole life in an increasingly scientific and technological age" (1960, p. 12). It is no surprise, then, that research quickly became the *raison d'etre* of graduate study—and remains so, despite continued criticism. Two other far-reaching characteristics of this period were (1) the application of the university's methods and training to the practical problems of society, and (2) specialization. There was insistence on making knowledge useful; the fruits of education were to be utilitarian and community centered. Further, specialization emerged as high school and undergraduate curricula were divided into subjects or disciplines similar to those in which the faculty had taken their graduate training, with the result that high school teachers, like the college professors who taught them, thought of themselves as historians or mathematicians rather than teachers (Berelson, 1960).

Between 1900 and World War I, higher education in the United States consolidated and became standardized while continuing its slow growth. Standardization was sought during this period for the procedures and programs of graduate study. The American Association of Universities (AAU) was founded in 1900 as the guardian of the values and practices of graduate study; its task being to set uniform standards for the PhD. In 1900 one-third of the PhDs awarded were for off-campus work or no work, and between eight and ten percent were honorary. Issues of frequent debate by the AAU during its early years are both useful and familiar: fellowships, the meaning of research, the character of the dissertation, the quality of the students, the foreign language requirement, the major–minor problem at the doctoral level, the proper examinations, the role of the master's, preparation for college teaching, college–university relations, uniform statistics. At the root of continued debate were the questions of the use of the doctorate, the meaning of the degree, the definition of the PhD, it's validity as a preparation for scholars or workers, whether it is a certificate of knowledge or a union card, and whether it results in proficiency or scholarship (Berelson, 1960). Standardization was constantly discussed, and those standards which eventually were accepted nationally and remain for the most part include: (1) having a baccalaureate degree, required for admission, (2) completing three years of postgraduate study, one of which must be in residency, (3) achieving foreign language proficiency, (4) taking general examinations, both written and oral, and (5) presenting an acceptable thesis (dissertation) characterized by original research and defended before the faculty (Walters, 1965). The honorary and off-campus PhDs were virtually nonexistent by World War I.

The period between World Wars I and II was marked by growth and diversification. Earned doctorates increased by over 500 percent during these years, and the number of institutions awarding the doctorate increased from 50 to nearly 100 (Berelson, 1960). It was during this time that "the composition of the graduate student body changed for good—away from whatever remained of the nineteenth century's genteel tradition and social elitism, toward primary concern with simple intellectual quality" (Berelson, 1960, p. 27). Moreover, choice of a field of doctoral study expanded to not only more specialized areas within the arts and sciences, but also the professional fields of agriculture, business, education, engineering, home economics, journalism, library science, social work, and finally, nursing. Growing specialization was also reflected in an expanding body of knowledge published in the scholarly and scientific literature. The number of scientific journals had increased from 1555 in the nineteenth century to 50,000 for less than half of the twentieth century (Berelson, 1960). The journals founded before 1900 tended to be generally applicable to each discipline; after 1900 they increasingly tended to focus on specialty and subspecialty areas.

There was great concern about the professions awarding any doctorate at all, but the PhD was especially disputed. Questions of purpose and quality surfaced again and were hotly debated. Should the PhD be awarded only for scholarship in the traditional arts and sciences? Should professional doctorates, e.g., EdD, D. Eng., DBA, DNS, be awarded for high achievement in the professions? The professions, generally, preferred the PhD—it symbolized that they had "arrived." Generally, the professions won; history supports that social pressures and funding most often win over "standards," the argument of the purists. Berelson (1960) points out that this was reminiscent of the struggle 50 years earlier when "the classics had argued against the entry of science on the grounds of inappropriate subject matter and method for 'true learning'"; and that in the current struggle the arts and sciences joined forces and used the old argument to try to keep out the professions (p. 28).

It is interesting to note that although the German model for PhD education brought to the United States was in a very real sense a professional degree, there were not job opportunities for doctorally-prepared workers outside of academe in the states. Because of this the PhD had to become more oriented toward pure learning than to professional training. By the time the United States was in need of and pressing for doctoral education as professional training, the "pure learning" tradition had been established and great resistance and controversy resulted from efforts to award the highest degree to those preparing for service (Harris, Troutt, & Andrews, 1980). In fact, Abraham Flexner's (1930), evaluation of the modern university severely criticized the American university for its service activities, calling them "service stations" for the general public.

Since World War II, growth and diversification have continued at an even greater rate. Three thousand doctorates were granted in 1952, a year which reflected World War II veterans returning to school on the GI bill. The most recent figures available indicate that 32,700 doctorates were awarded in 1987. Just as the number of graduates has increased dramatically, so has the number of fields in which doctoral training is offered; from approximately 450 fields in 1952, today 750 are available. The trend is toward increased numbers graduating from the professional fields at the expense of the humanities. However, there is a clear increase in the "professional" character of the work offered in the traditional academic disciplines, e.g., obtaining a doctorate in chemistry is excellent preparation for industrial practice or political science experts can work in public administration.

Despite the growth and change, the issues and the controversy, doctoral education in the United States has remained stable in several areas. Foremost is the preeminence of the PhD. Berelson points out that it is difficult to exaggerate the importance attached to the degree. "The exceptional regard that exists for the PhD in academic circles, where presumably most persons know better, has never been fully explained." Nearly everyone has preferred the PhD; other doctorates have always been accorded lower prestige. Berelson continues, "There can be no question . . . the 'magic' of the degree is among the most important legacies in the entire system" (1960, pp. 39–40).

Another stable characteristic of doctoral education is the primacy of research and training for research. The recipients of research training in one generation have become the faculty—the determiners of requirements in the next—so the traditions emerged and have been continued. However, this has led to charges, repeated over the years, that the graduate school is abnormally resistant to change.

Finally, the issues and controversies, the questions themselves, have remained stable. What does the PhD really mean? How can standards be maintained under the pressures of increasing numbers? Why aren't students better qualified? How many institutions should offer doctoral work? Should the professions award the PhD? *Plus ça change, plus c'est la même chose.*

THE PhD IN NURSING

The emergence of doctoral education in nursing began during the period of growth and diversification between the wars. In 1923, the Goldmark Report was published which carried recommendations regarding the development and strengthening of university schools of nursing. Although the response to the report appeared negligible, the number of nursing programs in institutions of higher learning slowly increased and, concomitantly, the need for better prepared nursing educators rose also. Although Teachers College, Columbia University, was the first institution in the United States to offer doctoral education in nursing (1924), it awarded an EdD with a major in administration or education, not a PhD. In 1934 New York University opened the first program leading to a PhD in nursing; it was offered in the School of Education and the majors were administration or education. The next program to offer the doctorate in nursing, another PhD, was the University of Pittsburgh in 1954. The major area of study was described as "nursing and related fields," i.e., child development, chemistry, administration, and education. Until this point, the growth of doctoral programs in nursing had been slow—one new program per decade. The next decade would see the beginning of the rapid growth that continues today.

After World War II when large numbers of nurses returned from the service desiring to use their GI Bill of Rights to earn a college degree, the number of nursing programs in institutions of higher learning increased rapidly, as did the demand for nursing educators with higher degrees. Consequently, master's nursing programs, particularly those preparing graduates for teaching, increased while the demand for doctorally-prepared nursing faculty rose in response. It is no surprise that education was the major most frequently pursued by these nursing faculty seeking doctoral preparation (Grace, 1978a). Murphy (1981), using Grace's work, further describes this first phase of doctoral education—1926 to 1959—as the phase of functional specialist preparation during which most doctoral degrees earned were in education: 47 PhD, 80 EdD, and 5 in other fields for a total of 132.

Grace (1978b) points out the key role that the federal government has played in influencing the direction of doctoral education in nursing, primarily through its funding initiatives. In 1955, the United States Public Health Service started funding doctoral study through the Federal Predoctoral Research Fellowship program. Funds were awarded directly to the doctoral student, and many aspiring faculty members were then able to pursue the doctorate. From 1955 through 1970, 156 nurses were supported by the Division of Nursing Fellowships.

Although the Faculty Research Development Grants Program (FaReDeGs) (begun in 1959) was developed to increase the research capability of faculty in graduate programs, the most frequent mode to accomplish this was funding for doctoral preparation. The grants also provided seed money for pilot studies. Eighteen institutions participated from 1959–1968 when the program was determined to have fulfilled its objectives and was phased out to be replaced by Research Development Grants. Of the 18, only 3 offered doctoral programs in nursing during the years of funding (1 PhD, 1 EdD, and 1 DNS), although 14 do now (10 PhD, 1 EdD, 2 DNS, and 1 PhD and DNS).

In 1962, in order to increase the research talent of nurses, the Division of Nursing, USPHS, funded doctoral study for nurses in other disciplines related to nursing. These were the Nurse Scientist Graduate Training Grants. According to Grace, the intent underlying the Nurse Scientist Program was to build a critical mass of faculty and create a receptive milieu for the development of doctoral programs in nursing (1978a). By 1973, 9 universities (34 departments) had received these grants, and 4 of the 9 universities then had doctoral programs in nursing: 2 PhD, 1 EdD, and 1 DNS. All nurse scientists earned PhDs; fields of study included sociology, psychology, anthropology, biology, and physiology.

In 1965 several nurse-scientist trainees and faculty at Case Western Reserve University invited four distinguished nurse leaders to speak at a symposium where they would address the different doctoral degree options available to nurses. Dr. Jeanne Berthold, moderator of the symposium, identified four issues related to doctoral preparation:

• What are the goals of doctoral preparation for nurses?

• Who are the "some nurses" who need to be prepared at the doctoral level in order to fulfill their role responsibilities adequately?

• What type of doctoral program should nurses undertake?

• When should a nurse be encouraged to go into a doctoral program? (1966a, p. 48)

Although all speakers agreed that the ultimate goal was the strong PhD in nursing, there was disagreement as to when the base of nursing science would support such a program. Two speakers agreed that the timing was not yet right for the PhD in nursing because nursing science in 1965 was not sufficiently developed to support the teaching research and scholarship needed for the PhD. Dr. Mary Tschudin (1966), Dean of Nursing at the University of Washington, instead spoke in support of an option utilized at her school—doctoral preparation for nurses through PhD programs in other disciplines with a minor in nursing. Education was the first to "open its doors," she reported, but over the years "sociology, anthropology, psychology, history, philosophy, microbiology, and physiology have accepted graduates of baccalaureate programs in nursing into their PhD programs" (p. 51). Dr. Rozella Schlotfeldt (1966), Dean of Nursing at Case Western Reserve University, expressed her position clearly: "Doctoral preparation leading to a PhD degree in a field of fundamental knowledge is the most useful and appropriate for a nurse . . . regardless of whether she plans to work primarily as a practitioner-investigator, as a practitioner-educator-investigator, or as an administrator of programs of nursing care or programs of nursing education" (p. 69).

Dr. Martha Rogers (1966), Chair of Nursing at New York University, differed with Tschudin and Schlotfeldt, believing that the time for the PhD in nursing was overdue. She was emphatic in her opinion that there was substantive baccalaureate and master's content in nursing and that the PhD was not a beginning, but an open-ended extension. Her program also offered a minor, but it was in a related science, not the other way around.

Dr. Hildegard Peplau (1966), Professor of Psychiatric Nursing at Rutgers University, developed the idea that there are two major career track options for graduate psychiatric nurses and pointed out that there are only two kinds of doctoral degrees in universities—the university degree (PhD) and the occupational degree (EdD, PharmD, DBA). With this in mind, she recommended that nurses choose a degree program to fit their ability and long range career plans. Dr. Peplau clarified the differences between the two degree options: the PhD prepares the graduate for clinical research and the derivation of new knowledge from the clinical data and the DNS prepares the graduate for expert nursing practice based on application of theory derived by others.

Murphy (1981) describes this second phase of doctoral study (1960-1969) as the nurse scientist era since so many nurses earned doctoral degrees in scientific disciplines related to nursing as well as in nursing—449 nurses earned 215 PhDs (nursing and non-nursing), 191 EdDs, and 43 other doctorates.

Murphy's (1981) third phase of doctoral education development—doctorates in and of nursing—was launched by the 1971 federally sponsored conference on *Future Directions of Doctoral Education for Nurses*. The conference was called to explore evolving trends in nursing education and identify the implications for federal funding of doctoral education for nursing. In particular, the Nurse Scientist Graduate Training Committee needed guidelines regarding the best type(s) of doctoral preparation for nurses so appropriate funding decisions could be made. The Division of Nursing invited four distinguished participants, two of whom had presented at the symposium at Case Western

Reserve University in 1965. Dr. Joseph Matarazzo (1971) presented a historical perspective of doctoral education and its implications for nursing. Rogers (1971) repeated her description of the PhD in nursing at NYU while Schlotfeldt (1971) again promoted the PhD in a scientific discipline related to nursing. Dr. Florence Erickson (1971) described a new concept, the clinical PhD. Because the invitational conference consisted of only 37 participants, there was opportunity for detailed discussion on the five major topic areas:

- Assessing nursing education needs

- The pluralistic approach to nursing education

- The research component in doctoral level education

- Expanding the Nurse Scientist Graduate Training Program

- Individual and institutional funding

Areas of general agreement were identified; most significant was the need for diversity in doctoral level nursing education in both the types of programs offered and the funding mechanisms developed to support them. Another need widely agreed upon was that of maintaining strong support for research preparation while expanding support for other types of nursing education.

Doctoral programs grew rapidly in the 1970s from 5 (1 EdD, 2 PhD, and 2 DNS) in 1970 to 22 (14 PhD, 1 EdD, and 7 professional degree) in 1980. Early in the decade there was rising concern about maintenance of quality in light of rapid expansion. Dr. Madeleine Leininger was requested by AACN to conduct a comprehensive survey of accredited schools offering graduate education in nursing ($n = 58$). Leininger (1976) identified several societal and professional forces that influenced the development of doctoral preparation for nurses and which still hold true:

- Changing role of women in our society

- The crisis in health care delivery

- The emergence of new types of health care facilities

- The need for research to examine nursing phenomena

- The need to change nursing education programs to fit societal imperatives

- The dissatisfaction of consumers with health care

The report of the survey (46 schools responded) was given at a 1974 national conference on issues in doctoral education for nurses. Leininger (1976) reported 7 existing doctoral programs in nursing and 6 for nursing; 22 were planned. She also reported on expected problems and issues that would likely emerge during the rapid growth period:

- Decreased and uncertain state and federal funding at a time of increased student interest in doctoral education in nursing

- Lack of well-prepared nursing administrators in service and education

- Essential features of nursing practice are not well-delineated

- The merits of different types of doctoral programs (research vs. practice) have not been clearly identified

The major concern was with the quality of existing and planned doctoral programs and the adequacy of the faculty in both numbers and preparation (Murphy, 1981). The major agreement of the conference group was the need for a National Planning Conference which could coordinate planning for doctoral programs in nursing (Leininger, 1976).

It is not clear whether the First National Conference on Doctoral Education in Nursing, held in 1977 for those presently offering or planning to initiate doctoral programs in nursing, was a direct response to the need identified at the 1974 conference, but the announced purpose suggests that it was. During her welcoming address Dr. Claire Fagin, Dean of the School of Nursing at the University of Pennsylvania, identified the essential need for the 1977 conference ". . . to consider components in planning, implementing and evaluating doctoral curriculum and to continue the development of a national information exchange of doctoral study in nursing" (p. 1).

Dr. Margaretta Styles' (1977) opening paper raised the question that had been the focus of the 1966 Conference at Case Western Reserve and one of the major questions addressed at the 1971 Future Directions Conference and the 1974 Issues Conference: Is there a difference between the PhD and the DNS? Is it real or imagined? Is it determined by principal or practicality? Conviction or compromise? Styles was very clear about the need to address and answer these questions:

. . . if I could, I would dump in the midst of us in this room the body of a putrefied, smelly dead jackass to remind us that we have left unsettled a fundamental question which cannot be avoided. We must sit in the presence of that stinking carcass until we have developed for the profession a rational, comprehensive, and definitive position on goal, program and degree differentiation. We cannot drift into hopeless confusion once again, we cannot further compound the confusion about nursing education which pervades our past and our very existence. If we were to become the principles, by design or default, in such a chapter in the history of the profession, we would leave a terrible legacy for our professional progeny and for society to untangle (p. 22).

The group agreed that degree title selection was most often decided by administrative policy, with approving committees and funding resources also exerting influence. Concerns were raised by the group regarding the wisdom of starting a new professional degree instead of using an established degree (PhD). One educator suggested starting with a DNS and eventually changing to the PhD, or changing the content to fit the PhD if the title could not be changed. Others believed that if the content and goals of programs with different titles were not clarified, it could "bastardize all degrees" (p. 86). The group decided that the conference had served a useful purpose and that they should meet again the following year.

This was the beginning of a tradition that continues to this day. Educators in existing and approved doctoral programs meet yearly, with one of the programs serving as host. The theme for the next forum is identified by a planning committee following the present year's conference based on suggestions from the attendees during the business meeting. The most relevant, significant, and scholarly topics are selected and appropriate speakers identified at the planning meeting.

The theme for the second forum was explication, description, and discussion of the various degree offerings. MacPhail (1978) described the new doctor of nursing program, Kelly (1978) the professional doctorate, and Grace (1978b) the research doctorate. Grace was explicit in her comparison of the goals of the two major doctorates: research—raise significant research questions in nursing as an applied scientific field; professional—prepare expert clinicians who may take the knowledge, apply it in the clinical setting, and test out the impact (1978b).

In 1984 the American Association of Colleges of Nursing (AACN) and the Division of Nursing sponsored a national invitational conference on doctoral education in nursing. The purposes were to reach consensus on issues of quality in doctoral programs in nursing, to define areas in which quality control is critical, to state criteria for assessing quality, and, to identify resources and relationships outside of the university which were crucial to the operation of such programs (Amos, 1984). Consensus statements were developed which related to faculty, program of study, resources, students, research, and evaluation of the programs. After the conference they were sent to participating schools for faculty review, reworked following that feedback, and broadly disseminated as indicators of quality. Following much debate regarding the PhD and DNS, the purposes of each, the lack of clarity between the two types of programs, and the wisdom of endorsing the PhD as the research degree and holding another similar conference to delineate the DNS, the conference participants decided that the indicators of quality would apply to both the PhD and the DNS (Watson, 1986).

Martin (1984), presenting the research doctorate in the debate at the Eighth Forum, reported on an analysis of program materials of 25 (19 PhD, 6 professional doctorate) existing doctoral programs (93% return). She found little to no difference between the research and professional degree programs. All programs emphasized nursing theory, statistics, and research. All required a minor and/or cognates and/or electives. All required the dissertation. The purpose statements varied little; all purported to prepare researchers and theoreticians who contribute to the body of knowledge. Preliminary to the presentation, Martin had distributed to the audience unidentified statements selected from the various program materials and requested that each statement be labeled as to the type of degree conferred by the program the purpose statement came from. When the instrument was scored it was clear that either the statements were not specific and clear or the audience did not know very much about doctoral education in nursing; the highest number correctly identified by any participant was 3 out of 12.

Although the topic of difference between the two degrees continued to be requested by some of the forum participants (usually by "new" members of the forum) for further discussion and debate, it has not been the focus of a forum or any major papers since 1984. It has been informally handled through designation as a breakfast or round table discussion topic. Those longstanding members of the forum who know the history of the topic and the relative lack of resolution which has followed even the most eloquent presentations may see continued debate as futile.

CONCLUSION

At this time the American Association of Colleges of Nursing has taken on the task. At an early 1988 Conference on Doctoral Education in Nursing, a motion was made from the floor that the conference go on record recommending that the PhD be *the* doctoral degree in nursing. The motion was never brought to vote, but a 1989 conference has been planned—A Position for Nursing in Doctoral Education: Consensus Building. The goals are to develop a position statement concerning doctoral education for nursing and to distinguish between the professional doctorate and the academic research doctorate. Clearly, if these goals are met, a great service will have been performed for the nursing profession. The questions which have echoed through the years since the professional doctorate became a reality (Berthold, 1966a; Matarazzo, 1971; Leininger, 1974; Styles, 1977; Grace, 1978b; Martin, 1984) would finally be answered.

Since the historical development of the PhD surely indicates that from its beginnings it has well served both academicians and practicing professionals, we are left to question why the need exists to complicate nursing's already difficult progression to full acceptance in the university and workplace. The PhD is the most appropriate degree for nursing, if nursing wishes to take its place as one of the respected scholarly disciplines. In addition, it is the most highly valued degree, allowing the widest range of employment possibilities.

Since 1980 the number of doctoral programs has more than doubled again (22 to 47); it had quadrupled from 1970 to 1980 (5 to 22). Of more interest to this topic, the ratio between the numbers of research and professional programs, which was 2:1 in 1970 and 1980, has shifted to nearly 3:1. Perhaps, as was suggested in 1984, because there are few real differences between the two types of programs, the shift or movement is toward one type of doctoral program in nursing—the PhD. (Martin). It is time for nursing leaders to learn from the past, make the difficult decisions in the present, to ensure the best future for the profession.

REFERENCES

Amos, L. (1984). Forward. *Proceedings of doctoral programs in nursing—Consensus for quality*. Washington, DC: American Association of Colleges of Nursing.

Ben-David, J. (1977). *Center of learning*. New York: McGraw-Hill.

Berelson, B. (1960). *Graduate education in the United States*. New York: McGraw-Hill.

Berthold, J. (1966a). A dialogue on approaches to doctoral preparation. *Nursing Forum, 5*(2), 48–49.

Berthold, J. (1966b). Panel discussion. *Nursing Forum, 5*(2), 83–108.

Brodie, B. (1986). Impact of doctoral programs on nursing education. *Journal of Professional Education, 2*(6), 350–357.

Fagin, C. (1977). Introductory remarks. In *First National Conference on Doctoral Education in Nursing* (pp. 1–2). Philadelphia: University of Pennsylvania School of Nursing.

Fields, W. (1988). The PhD: The ultimate nursing doctorate. *Nursing Outlook, 36*(4), 188–189.

Flexner, A. (1930). *Universities: American, English, German*. New York: Oxford University Press.

Goldmark, J. (1923). *Nursing and Nursing Education in the United States*. New York: Macmillan.

Grace, H. (1978a). The development of doctoral education in nursing: In historical perspective. *Journal of Nursing Education, 17*(4), 17–27.

Grace, H. (1978b). The research doctorate in nursing. In *Proceedings of the 1978 Forum on Doctoral Education in Nursing* (pp. 40–59). Chicago: Rush University.

Group Discussion. (1977). In *First National Conference on Doctoral Education in Nursing* (pp. 85–87a). Philadelphia: University of Pennsylvania School of Nursing.

Harris, J., Troutt, W., & Andrews, G. (1980). *The American doctorate in the context of new patterns in higher education*. Washington, DC: Council on Post Secondary Accreditation.

Kelly, J. (1978). The professional doctorate in nursing from the viewpoint of nursing service. In *Proceedings of the 1978 Forum on Doctoral Education in Nursing* (pp. 10–39). Chicago: Rush University.

Lash, A. (1987). The nature of the Doctor of Philosophy degree: Evolving conceptions. *Journal of Professional Nursing, 3*(2), 92–101.

Leininger, M. (1976). Doctoral programs for nurses: A survey of trends, issues and projected developments. In *The Doctorally Prepared Nurse* (DHEW Publication No. HRA 76-18, pp. 3-53). Bethesda, MD: U.S. Department of Health, Education and Welfare.

MacPhail, J. (1978). Doctor of nursing program: The professional doctorate in nursing. In *Proceedings of the 1978 Forum on Doctoral Education in Nursing* (pp. 1-9). Chicago: Rush University.

Martin, E. J. (1984). The research doctorate. In *Proceedings of the Eighth National Forum on Doctoral Education in Nursing* (pp. 1-9). Denver: University of Colorado School of Nursing.

Matarazzo, J. (1971). Perspective. In *Future Directions of Doctoral Education for Nurses: Report of a Conference* (pp. 49-105). Bethesda, MD: U.S. Department of Health, Education and Welfare.

Matarazzo, J., & Abdellah, F. (1971). Doctoral education for nurses in the United States. *Nursing Research, 20*(5), 404-414.

Murphy, J. (1981). Doctoral education in, of, and for nursing: An historical analysis. *Nursing Outlook, 29*(11), 645-649.

The Oxford English Dictionary, The Compact Edition. (1971). Oxford, England: Oxford University Press.

Peplau, H. (1966). Nursing: Two routes to doctoral degrees. *Nursing Forum, 5*(2), 57-67.

Rogers, M. (1966). Doctoral education in nursing. *Nursing Forum, 5*(2), 75-82.

Rogers, M. (1971). PhD in nursing. In *Future Directions of Doctoral Education for Nurses: Report of a Conference* (pp. 106-118). Bethesda, MD: U.S. Department of Health, Education and Welfare.

Rubin, R. and Erickson, F. (1971). Clinical doctorate. In *Future Directions of Doctoral Education for Nurses: Report of a Conference* (pp. 144-157). Bethesda, MD: U.S. Department of Health, Education and Welfare.

Schlotfeldt, R. (1966). Doctoral study in basic disciplines: A choice for nurses. *Nursing Forum, 5*(2), 68-74.

Schlotfeldt, R. (1971). PhD in science. In *Future Directions of Doctoral Education for Nurses: Report of a Conference* (pp. 120-142). Bethesda, MD: U.S. Department of Health, Education and Welfare.

Spurr, S. H. (1970). *Academic degree structure: Innovative approaches.* New York: McGraw-Hill.

Storr, R. (1953). *The beginnings of graduate education in America.* Chicago: University of Chicago Press.

Styles, M. (1977). Doctoral education in nursing: The current situation in historical perspective. In *First National Conference on Doctoral Education in Nursing* (pp. 3-24). Philadelphia: University of Pennsylvania School of Nursing.

Tschudin, M. (1966). Doctoral preparation in other disciplines: With a minor in nursing. *Nursing Forum, 5*(2), 50–56.

Walters, E. (Ed.). (1965). *Graduate education today.* Washington, DC: American Council on Education.

Watson, J. (1986). *Memorandum regarding position statement: Indicators of quality in doctoral programs in nursing.* Washington, DC: American Association of Colleges of Nursing.

2

The Doctor of Nursing Science Degree: Evolutionary and Societal Perspectives

Sr. Mary Jean Flaherty, PhD, RN, FAAN

BACKGROUND

The first Doctor of Nursing Science (DNS) degree was awarded by Boston University to Gertrude Isaacs. The program was inaugurated in 1960 with psychiatric nursing as the clinical area of study (American Journal of Nursing, 1963; Editorials, 1963). Dr. Isaacs completed a program of study in nursing that was augmented by a community mental health program at Harvard University where she was a special studies student. Her program reflected the ambiguity about what constituted doctoral study in nursing in the early 1960s. It also frames the problems of writing about evolutionary and societal perspectives on the Doctor of Nursing Science degree (DNS).

The initials DNS are used throughout this chapter to designate all DNS, DNSc, and DSN programs. The DNS was defined at the 1984 Conference on Doctoral Programs in Nursing as the professional degree that "emphasizes advanced clinical practice with integration of research to improve nursing care" (Jamann, 1985, p. 92). This definition is compatible with the American Nurses' Association (ANA) (1981) definition which promotes the DNS degree as an advanced clinical practice degree that integrates new knowledge into nursing care.

The literature of doctoral education yields very little about DNS programs. These programs have been referred to as professional degrees by Amos in 1985, Andreoli in 1987, Cleland in 1976, Jamann in 1985, Lash in 1987, Leininger in 1976, Murphy in 1984, and Snyder-Halpern in 1986. They are described as clinical degrees by Abdellah in 1966, Christman in 1978, Forni

17

and Welch in 1987, and Grace in 1978. In 1966 Peplau called the DNS an occupational degree in nursing.

Although the DNS is most often described as a clinical practice degree, some PhD nursing programs, such as the one offered at The University of Pittsburgh (Division of Nursing, 1971), also report heavy emphasis on advanced clinical practice. When clinical issues in doctoral nursing programs are discussed in the literature it is not always clear whether the reference is to the professional DNS or the academic PhD degree program. Ambiguity in the literature about the nature of the two degrees reflects a lack of consensus and a continuing debate among nursing leaders about the appropriate degree designation for doctoral programs in nursing (Andreoli, 1987; Cleland, 1976; Curran, Habeeb, & Sobel, 1981; Division of Nursing, 1971; Downs, 1978; Forni & Welch, 1987; Elkins, 1960; Lambertson, 1976). There is agreement, however, about the fact that two types of degree programs are needed and that one of them should be the DNS. Leininger (1976b) contended that healthy debates and research were needed to decide the best direction for emerging doctoral programs in nursing.

In recent years, however, many more PhD than DNS programs have been developed so that currently there are 33 PhD programs, 12 DNS programs, and 1 EdD program (National League for Nursing, 1987). Table 1 presents DNS programs currently being offered. Among schools that were planning doctoral programs in 1987, 36 intended to initiate PhD programs and 7 the DNS program (Andreoli, 1987). These figures, as well as the literature (Andreoli, 1987; Curran et al., 1981; Brimmer, Skoner, Pender, Williams, Fleming, & Werley, 1983; Murphy, 1985), indicate that the PhD program in nursing is presently favored by administrators, faculty, and students. This phenomenon raises some important questions. Why did the DNS degree originate? Does the degree

TABLE 1.   Current programs offering the professional degree.

School	Degree
University of Alabama	DSN
Boston University*	DNS
State University of New York (SUNY)/Buffalo	DNS
The Catholic University of America	DNSc
University of California/San Francisco	DNS
University of California/Los Angeles	DNSc
University of San Diego	DNS
Rush University	DNSc
Indiana University	DNS
Louisiana State University	DNS
Widener University	DNSc
George Mason University	DNSc

National League for Nursing. (1987). *Doctoral programs in nursing 1986–1987.* New York: National League for Nursing.
*This program has since closed.

designation make a difference in program content and focus? Why is there now such a skewed preference for the PhD program in nursing?

EVOLUTIONARY PERSPECTIVES: WHY THE DNS DEGREE?

The evolution of Doctor of Nursing Science programs has generally followed the pattern of nursing education in the twentieth century. It has been accompanied by intensive debate among nursing leaders, a lack of confidence in the credibility of the degree, and confusion about appropriate program content.

A review and analysis of 3 national meetings on doctoral education in nursing that were held over a 20-year span will highlight the issues related to the evolution of the DNS programs. The first meeting was a symposium held on May 19, 1965 under the auspices of the Francis Payne Bolton School of Nursing of Western Reserve University and reported in *Nursing Forum* (Berthold, 1966). The aim of this meeting, considered to be a watershed in the evolution of doctoral programs in nursing, was to provide a forum for "a scholarly discussion of the strengths and problems inherent in the various approaches to doctoral education for nurses" (Berthold, 1966, p. 49). Four issues framed the organization of the symposium: (a) the goals of doctoral preparation for nurses; (b) identification of nurses to be educated; (c) type of doctoral program; and (d) the appropriate time for nurses to begin doctoral study. Four leaders, Hildegard Peplau, Rozella Schlotfeldt, Martha Rogers, and Mary Tschudin, presented their views on the issues.

Peplau (1966) believed that nurses should have the opportunity to select, based on their ability and long-range goals, either the PhD university degree, the EdD degree, or the DNS degree (which she termed the occupational degree). Peplau stated that the DNS candidate would pursue in-depth clinical training and would have exposure to research methods. A dissertation would be required but it would not be an original study leading to new knowledge. The DNS graduate would be involved in the testing of existing theories and the application of knowledge discovered by others, some of it "hot off the press" (Peplau, 1966, p. 66). Peplau was careful to point out that this approach to doctoral education in nursing did not preclude the possibility that some original findings might be discovered by DNS-prepared nurses.

Schlotfeldt (1966), on the other hand, was a strong proponent of nurses obtaining their PhD in disciplines other than nursing. She argued that multidisciplinary knowledge was needed in nursing; that it was impossible for one person to become a scholar in all required areas and that nurses prepared in the basic disciplines had more freedom to explain nursing problems and to profit from collaboration with other scientists. Her position in support of the PhD degree for nurses was reinforced by Rogers (1966) who argued that the PhD should be in nursing because basic research was needed before applied research could be initiated. Rogers was concerned about the use of the term "clinical research" by some nursing programs, believing that it signified applied research. Tschudin (1966) discussed the merits of obtaining the PhD in another discipline such as sociology, anthropology, psychology, or philosophy, with a minor in nursing. She pointed out that the first nurses who graduated from these programs did not return to nursing. This view, however, was refuted by Abdellah (1966), citing USPHS statistics which indicated that of 150 predoctoral nurse fellows graduated by 1966, 90 percent were employed in nursing education, service, or consultation.

In the continuing dialogue about doctoral study, other leaders responded to the papers presented at the symposium. The need for two kinds of doctorates, the academic PhD and the professional DNS, was a predominant theme, but the lack of differentiation between them was viewed as a major problem. For instance, Nahm (1966) wrote that, whether the earned degree was a PhD in nursing or the DNS, advanced preparation and research in nursing had to form the core of both programs, suggesting that they had common goals. Adding to the confusion, Kemble (1966) argued that there was room for diversity in doctoral nursing programs without necessarily creating divisiveness.

Others (Hadley, 1966; Hassenplug, 1966) contended that existing doctoral programs were not truly nursing doctorates, whether PhD or DNS. They believed that nursing had not yet identified what constituted nursing knowledge or science (Hadley, 1966) or that the nursing content had not been delineated sufficiently to distinguish the clinical nursing doctorate (Hassenplug, 1966). In her response to the symposium report, Abdellah (1966) suggested that the PhD in the behavioral or hard sciences was the better doctoral training at a time when professional nursing was developing toward maturity. She thought that although the DNS programs held promise, they were too new to evaluate. Abdellah emphasized the emerging role of the clinical specialist that she identified with the DNS program. However, she used Boston University (DNS) and University of Pittsburgh (PhD) as examples of doctoral programs in clinical nursing.

The 1971 conference was sponsored and assembled by the Division of Nursing at Bethesda, Maryland in January of 1971 and reported in *Future Directions of Doctoral Education for Nurses*. This meeting assisted the Nurse Scientist Training Committee in its work with schools of nursing that were funded for PhD programs for nurse scientists (Division of Nursing, 1971). Although the conference discussion centered on the need for clinical studies at the doctoral level, the major focus of the conference was on the development of PhD programs in nursing, while the DNS programs were rarely mentioned. The lack of emphasis on the development of the DNS programs was notable because one of the three issues identified for discussion at the conference was "How can a balance between clinical nursing and clinical research be achieved within a Doctor of Nursing Science degree?" (Division of Nursing, 1971, p. viii).

Conference members agreed that the PhD was the preferred program by most students, faculty, and leaders in scientific disciplines; that DNS programs should focus on applications of new knowledge; and that the Nurse Scientist Graduate Training Program, which funded doctoral level programs in disciplines other than nursing, should be expanded to include doctoral level nursing programs. This latter recommendation included both DNS and PhD programs.

The third conference, sponsored jointly by the Division of Nursing and the American Association of Colleges of Nursing and summarized in *Proceedings of Doctoral Programs in Nursing: Consensus for Quality* in 1984, concentrated on the promotion and maintenance of quality in existing and developing doctoral programs in nursing (Jamann, 1985). Doctoral programs had expanded from 9 in 1974 to 30 in 1984 with 7 of these programs leading to the DNS degree. Jamann (1985) predicted that because of economic constraints within higher education, the growth of doctoral programs in nursing would slow in the 1980s, even though the need for them was no longer an issue.

During the conference Amos (1985) reviewed the continuing debate on the nature, title of the degree, and the distinguishing characteristics of each program. She reminded the audience of several salient factors: that the 1984 Doctoral Forum had found little or no differences between existing doctoral programs and that it was no longer possible for programs to prepare both researchers and clinical doctors of nursing. Finally, she recommended that a set of criteria be designed specifically for the PhD and the DNS programs in order to distinguish between them.

In the ensuing discussion led by Chioni, it was pointed out that while there was a need for differentiation between programs, the focus of the DNS programs was less clear than it was for the PhD programs. Some participants expressed an interest in a future conference to study the entry-level ND and the advanced DNS programs. Others raised questions about the wisdom of seeking differentiation between programs, pleading rather for agreement that the PhD program should be the program for nursing in the future.

It is clear from these three conferences as well as the literature (Andreoli, 1987; Amos, 1985; Curran et al., 1981; Grace, 1978a; Lancaster, 1985; Lash, 1987; Murphy, 1984, 1985; Shores, 1986; Snyder-Halpern, 1986) that the differences between DNS and PhD programs has not been resolved. It is also clear that DNS programs are not accorded equal respect among nursing leaders. Nor has federal funding been as readily available for the development of DNS programs over the past 20 years. And, although there was general support for both PhD and DNS programs at the 1984 conference, participants expressed the desire to have a statement developed by the American Association of Colleges of Nursing that would clarify the future of doctoral education in nursing. Grace (1978c) summarized the issue when she wrote:

> Considerable controversy surrounds the nature of doctoral education in nursing. First and foremost, nurse educators hold differing views on the nature of research and theory development in nursing, with some viewing nursing as a pure science and others arguing that nursing is an applied field (p. 118).

She suggested that although two types of doctoral programs in nursing, professional and academic, were needed and were in place in 1978, program objectives and end products were not clearly differentiated. She argued for the:

> . . . development of a cadre of doctorally prepared nurses in clinical practice who are expert clinicians, but who also have a grounding in research enabling them to test out the effects of clinical interventions within the patient care setting, be it hospital, home, or community. With such a group of doctorally prepared nurses, it is at last possible to conceptualize the movement of the profession to a place of stature in its own right (Grace, 1978c, p. 121).

Yet even before Grace's assessment of doctoral nursing programs in 1978, there was controversy and debate about the appropriate degree offerings in nursing. Earlier Matarazzo (Division of Nursing, 1971) mused on nursing's past history that he characterized as "often chaotic and emotion laden" (p. 64). He pointed out that nursing was in a parallel position with other applied disciplines—education, fine arts, applied mathematics, and psychology—in their attempt to establish curricula at the doctoral level, but that these programs had agreed on a pattern of doctoral education one to five decades earlier. This lack of consensus about the appropriate degree resulted in four types of doctorates in nursing being offered in 1971: the Doctor of Nursing (DN), Doctor of Nursing Science (DNS or DNSc), Doctor of Nursing Education (DNEd), and Doctor of Public Health Nursing (DPhN). Matarazzo blamed this disagreement about the preferred degree on developments of the previous decade involving nurses themselves, the major nursing organizations (ANA and NLN), university faculties, and the federal government. Heidgerken (1973) believed the lack of consensus to be a reason for the reluctance of educators to develop doctoral programs in nursing. She explained and defended the initiation of a DNS program at The Catholic University of America because:

> . . . the profession has reached the period in its development when it is compelled by its obligation to society to develop a program of doctoral study. The proportion of responsibility for health care which professional nurses are asked to carry has increased markedly in recent decades . . . profession must provide personnel who can exercise a creative leadership that is analytical and scholarly in clinical nursing, teaching and administration (p. 12).

However, others (Amos, 1985; Cleland, 1976; Grace, 1983) challenged the belief by many nurses that they, unlike those in other disciplines, must be all things—teacher, practitioner, and researcher. By 1978 Grace was calling for research on the question of whether it was possible to prepare graduates of a doctoral program with the skills of both researcher and clinician:

> Until such a time as this question is addressed, it appears that there is a critical need for doctorally prepared nurses in clinical practice settings that are engaged in

modification of practice as their primary goal. For want of a better term, I would characterize nurses in such positions as the "social engineers" of the patient care system, whose function is that of taking knowledge generated by nurse researchers and testing it out within a broader clinical context. Currently, I do not see such a doctoral program model clearly delineated . . . (Grace, 1978b p. 26).

Five years later Grace (1983) described a proposed curriculum model for a two-track, four-year doctoral program in nursing. Common core courses would be offered to professional and research track students in the first year. Clinical practicum experiences for professional students were designed so that they would become highly proficient in a clinical specialty area. At the end of the second year the MSN degree would be awarded. Third and fourth year professional students would become increasingly specialized with clinical seminars and practica. Fourth year students would do an internship experience and design a clinical research study, the purpose of which was to give them the opportunity to show their competency to apply knowledge in the practice arena. Grace (1983) assumed that students in both tracks would elect courses in the functional areas of nursing, teaching, and administration.

The structure of the doctoral programs in nursing was relatively easy to design. The fabric or content of the programs was much more difficult to define. During the 1970s while it was believed that the professional clinical doctorate should focus on clinical specialization (Grace, 1978b; Cleland, 1976), this did not occur in the curricula as designed at that time. By 1988 Downs was still calling for less attention to the structure of doctoral programs and more emphasis on the content.

Concern about the content of doctoral programs led Leininger (1976a) to blame the critical shortage of nurse educators, administrators, and researchers on the heavy emphasis placed on clinical specialists to address those leadership needs. Grace (1978a) raised another issue regarding the clinical component built into many programs. She acknowledged that it was the most difficult content to define and distinguish from the master's level and suggested that:

> This is perhaps an outgrowth of the difficulty of theory building in an applied field; the clinician is not merely an expert technician but must also build clinical knowledge as part of practice . . . The challenge in professional doctoral degree programs with a clinical focus is to move nursing theory from a descriptive level to one of intervention and then to build an analysis of the effects of intervention into the knowledge base of the practice profession (Grace, 1978a, p. 80).

Not only was the clinical component difficult to distinguish from master's level study, but some believed that it was the least well developed in doctoral education (Division of Nursing, 1971; Grace, 1978a; Hassenplug, 1966; Lash, 1987).

Matarazzo and Abdellah (1971) argued that the PhD would generate new knowledge and the DNS would apply it. Studies have demonstrated, however, that there were few noticeable differences between program types (Holzemer, 1987; Lancaster, 1985; Snyder-Halpern, 1986) and that programs tended to be more alike than different. Beare, Gray, and Ptak (1981) examined the content of existing doctoral nursing programs and concluded that the programs were preparing scholars and researchers rather than leaders in education and administration urged by Leininger (1976b).

Although Holzemer (1987) did not distinguish between doctoral programs in his study of quality indicators, his findings suggested that all programs experienced considerable growth between 1979 and 1984. He reported greater faculty commitment to scholarly work and an increase in students admitted to doctoral study with improved academic credentials. He concluded that there was a growing maturity in all doctoral programs in nursing as far as their scholarly climates were concerned, implying few differences between program types.

Lancaster (1985) compared the philosophy, objectives, and nature of dissertations for 14 PhD and 6 DNS programs. He found a blurring of the nature of the programs, but observed that the philosophy and objectives statements of the DNS programs were more consistent with the identified characteristics than were those of the PhD programs. He reported that:

> None of the DNS programs stated a focus that was characteristic of a PhD. All of the DNS programs believed that the primary focus was related to inquiry into nursing practice to improve health care delivery, to prepare professional practitioners, and to prepare expert clinicians who modify nursing practice (Lancaster, 1985, p. 59).

In her study of four PhD and four DNS programs, Snyder-Halpern (1986) also found that there were more curricular similarities than differences between them. She reported that the most differences were found in the areas of program purposes and objectives. One PhD program and all four DNS programs identified the preparation of clinicians as a primary program purpose and all four PhD and one DNS program reported that the preparation of researchers was the main focus.

In a study of 22 doctoral programs admitting students between 1981 and 1982, Murphy (1985) found no differentiation among philosophy, objectives, and conceptual frameworks between professional and research degrees. In her exhaustive review of the historical, program, outcome, and product studies on doctoral programs in nursing reported between 1950 and the 1980s, she concluded that "the degree designation did not reflect accurately the type of program in which the nurse was involved" (Murphy, 1985, p. 186).

Since the differences between the two degree programs appears to be so slight the question emerges about why there have been so few DNS programs developed in recent years. Professional self-image and concern about the respect other disciplines have for nursing may be among the reasons. Elkins (1960), for instance, wrote that "the doctorate should not be established as a minimum requirement unless it is designed to serve a real purpose, and this purpose should not be merely to raise the prestige of nursing" (p. 544). She believed that the nursing doctorate should be offered by a few schools with strong undergraduate programs and pleaded for nursing "to devise a plan for the future that will command the respect of the professions and the generous support of the public whose interests are paramount" (p. 544). McManus (1960) also warned against the initiation of doctoral programs in nursing to raise the prestige of nursing. Later, Matarazzo (Division of Nursing, 1971) identified two principal reasons for nursing's initial hesitation in plunging into doctoral education: self-concept and the overly romanticized view that nurses have of the scientific process. In the 1971 conference he was recorded as saying:

> In articles, debates, and conferences, nurses engaged in agonizing soul-searching and stock-taking about practice derived from principle and scientific theory in its relation to practice. These articles read like sophomore level text books . . . They are nonsense and a wasteful exercise. Nurses talk and talk and talk about science instead of doing it (Division of Nursing, 1971, pp. 9–10).

Science according to Matarazzo had little relationship to practice, a fact that he found true for all disciplines. He questioned why nursing thought it was different from the others. By 1978 Grace was warning that "It is time that nursing move away from its sexist self-identity problem and assume full responsibility and authority as equal partners in the health care arena" (Grace, 1978b, p. 27). The warning by Grace certainly extended to nursing's attempt to fit into the academic world, (especially in the evolution of doctoral study) that has continued to be a source of frustration. Downs, writing in 1978, pointed out that:

> . . . the university community tends to share the public's image of nursing as a technically and medically oriented occupation without a free-standing or substantive knowledge base. They do not understand, for instance, why degrees in other fields do not meet our needs let alone know and understand that we have already gone that route and found it lacking (p. 60).

Christman (1978) identified an image problem associated with lack of doctoral preparation and clinical research among faculty members. As a result nursing was not perceived as a true profession and nurses were not appointed to the influential policymaking committees on campus. Although he supported the clinical doctorate, he acknowledged that nurses with earned doctorates in cognate fields of science were in better strategic positions within the academic community. Cleland (1976) offered a slightly different view of the relationship between the academic community and nurses with professional or clinical degrees. She recommended that persons with professional degrees should be employed as clinical or adjunct faculty or lecturers because most of them could not meet the requirements for research and scholarly activities required by major research universities. She concluded that the professional degree would not be the best preparation for faculty because it would not be recognized by other schools. She wrote:

Medicine, years ago, found that it could not provide the training for advanced clinical practice within the framework of the university's value system, or operationalized in the course credit and tenure systems . . . If medicine, with its tremendous societal-based power, could not set aside the university's value system, which rewards the creation of knowledge rather than skill development, why should nursing make such an attempt? Nursing, for full acceptance by universities, must have academically qualified faculty members prepared to envelop new knowledge in support of the university's goals (Cleland, 1976, p. 632).

Downs (1978) in responding to these remarks, disputed Cleland's assessment. She pointed out the need to distinguish between the DN and DNS: the DN would be likened to the MD degree, and the DNS graduate would be prepared for university teaching. She concluded that ". . . it is imperative that the nursing profession straighten out this potential morass" (p. 59).

Murphy (1981) also noted that there was a growing concern that nurses have not been recognized as colleagues in both the academic and practice settings. She raised important questions about this phenomenon.

The constantly distracting puzzlement has to do with our knowledge base. Is it unique so that we can claim professional status? Is it scientific? Does it serve as the rationale for practice? Has it been derived through the process of scientific inquiry? (p. 649)

She concluded that analysis of current doctoral education "for, in, and of nursing is needed to address the questions" (p. 649).

By 1987, Andreoli would still note that the debate about the appropriate degree for nursing had raged for years, and that it centered around which projects the better image and had more credibility in academic settings. Certainly, she argued that the PhD was a credential which was well established in scientific and academic communities; that it did most to enhance the image of nurses; that it made it easier for nursing faculty to achieve tenure; and that the recent trend for increased nursing research added to the move toward the research PhD. However, she proposed another curricular model which combined the DSN/PhD. It is important to note that she was recommending the DSN, not DNS, a distinction that she believed was critical. Her arguments for proposing this model were based on several theses. First, nursing needed to make a clear statement to other health professionals and health care consumers about the nature of the scientific base of nursing. Next, the DSN followed logically from the MSN. Finally, if the degree was a DNS, it implied that nursing was a science in itself while it was actually still in the early stages of development. Therefore, the preferred degree should be the DSN.

Grace (1983) also acknowledged that self-esteem plagued nursing as a problem in the development of doctoral programs in nursing. She referred to this as the "Avis" or "We try harder" phenomenon in our attempts to be everything and observed that:

This is evidenced by our holding to the belief that all nurses can and should do everything equally well. Assuming that nurses can be researchers, expert clinicians, and teachers simultaneously imposes a burden found in very few other academic disciplines . . . In nursing, we need both our scholar-theoretician and our performing artists, the clinicians. And most certainly, there needs to be carefully constructed communication between groups lest they begin to track off in different directions, thus producing a cacophony (Grace, 1983, p. 151).

The concern about the best degree to possess also infiltrated the literature on the selection of a doctoral program by prospective students. For example, Curran, et al. (1981) warned that the PhD and EdD degree programs were well established in the scientific and academic communities while the DNS was not. Prospective students should ask how important a specific degree was to their self-esteem. They argued that "nursing, like all other groups, attaches importance to symbols. Degrees from all of the programs may serve the same function in the job market, but in terms of prestige, they may not be interchangeable" (p. 37).

DISCUSSION

The cacophony identified by Grace has been present over the years as the DNS programs evolved. While many leaders in nursing proclaimed the merit of having two tracks in doctoral education in nursing, little was done to delineate clearly the differences that should be present between them. It is obvious that the PhD research track is the degree preferred by universities, faculties, and students even though there has also been consensus and continuing discussions about the need for doctorally prepared nurses with strong clinical knowledge and skills. One can speculate as to why this has occurred.

Certainly a major reason is the ever present concern about the identity and image of nursing, especially within the academic community. All too often there are comparisons by nursing faculty as to whether their knowledge base is as scientific, as important, as scholarly as that of other disciplines. Because nurses allow this to occur among themselves, it is easily communicated to other faculties so that a vicious cycle of self-doubt and confirmation of that doubt occurs. Several years ago, in one nursing school that offers a DNS degree, there was some discussion about changing to a PhD program. During informal discussions about the advisability of making the change, a frequently asked question was, "Could the change in degree be retroactive?", that is, "Could my DNS be converted to a PhD?" If one thinks about this, it raises serious questions about the value placed on the outward symbol, in this case, the name of the degree, rather than on the knowledge and skill that the degree represents.

Despite the controversy that continues to exist it is clear that DNS programs prepare clinically strong, well-educated nurses who can set new directions, manage nursing systems, educate future nurses, and control the quality of nursing services in the health care system. The clinical professional doctorate (DNS) is one model of education that provides the essential knowledge and skills to ensure that these nurses are available. The initiation of these programs has been done in good faith and in response to societal needs. It appears however that the DNS programs continue to be viewed as less desirable than PhD programs by many students, faculty, and nurse administrators. Clearly it is time for the profession to either confirm the appropriateness of the DNS degree or to designate the preferred doctoral degree in nursing. If more value were accorded to DNS programs by the profession, those who earn the degree would have more pride in what they have accomplished and in what they are contributing to the profession of nursing and to the health care of society.

REFERENCES

Abdellah, F. G. (1966). Doctoral preparation for nurses: A continuation of the dialogue. *Nursing Forum, 3*, 44–53.

American Journal of Nursing. (1963). Boston's first Doctorate in Nursing Science goes to nurse-midwife. *American Journal of Nursing, 63*(8), 27.

American Nurses' Association. (1981). *Nurses with earned doctorates.* Kansas City, MO: American Nurses' Association.

Amos, L. K. (1985). Issues in doctoral preparation in nursing: Current perspectives and future directions. *Journal of Professional Nursing, 1*, 101–121.

Andreoli, K. G. (1987). DSN: Specialization and graduate curricula: Finding the fit. *Nursing and Health Care, 8*(2), 65–69.

Beare, P. G., Gray, C. J., & Ptak, H. F. (1981). Doctoral curricula in nursing. *Nursing Outlook, 29*, 311–316.

Berthold, J. S. (1966). Approaches to doctoral preparation for nurses. A dialogue on approaches to doctoral preparation [Introduction]. *Nursing Forum, 5*(2), 48–56.

Brimmer, P. F., Skoner, R. M. M., Pender, N. J., Williams, C. A., Fleming, J. W., & Werley, H. H. (1983). Nurses with doctoral degrees: Education and employment characteristics. *Research in Nursing and Health, 6*(4), 157–165.

Christman, L. (1978). Doctoral education: A shot in the arm for the nursing profession. *Nursing Digest, 6*(2), 45.

Cleland, J. (1976, October). Developing a doctoral program . . . Wayne State University, Detroit. *Nursing Outlook, 24*, 631–635.

Curran, C. L., Habeeb, M. C., & Sobol, E. G. (1981). Selecting a doctoral program for a career in nursing. *Journal of Nursing Administration, 11*, 35–40.

Division of Nursing. (1971). *Future directions of doctoral education for nurses* (DHEW Publication No. (NIH) 72-82). Washington, DC: U. S. Department of Health, Education and Welfare.

Downs, F. S. (1978, January). Doctoral education in nursing: Future directions. *Nursing Outlook, 26,* 56-61.

Downs, F. S. (1988). Doctoral education: Our claim to the future. *Nursing Outlook, 36*(1), 18-20.

Editorials. (1963, July 11). First doctor of nursing science. *New England Journal of Medicine, 269,* 109-110.

Elkins, W. H. (1960, October). Doctoral education in nursing: A university president presents his point of view. *Nursing Outlook, 8,* 542-544.

Forni, P. R., & Welch, M. J. (1987). The professional versus the academic model: A dilemma for nursing education. *Journal Professional Nursing, 3*(5), 291-297.

Grace, H. K. (1978a). Doctoral education: Past, present and future. In J. A. Williamson (Ed.), *Current perspectives in nursing education,* (Vol. 2) (pp. 72-89). St. Louis: C. V. Mosby.

Grace, H. K. (1978b, April). The development of doctoral education in nursing: An historical perspective. *Journal Nursing Education, 17,* 17-27.

Grace, H. K. (1978c). The development of doctoral education in nursing: An historical perspective. In N. L. Chaska (Ed.), *The nursing profession: Views through the mist* (pp. 112-123). New York: McGraw-Hill.

Grace, H. K. (1983). Doctoral education in nursing: Dilemmas and directions. In N. L. Chaska (Ed.), *The nursing profession: A time to speak* (pp. 144-155). New York: McGraw-Hill.

Hadley, B. J. (1966). Doctoral preparation for nurses: A continuation of the dialogue. *Nursing Forum, 3,* 59-60.

Hassenplug, L. W. (1966). Doctoral preparation for nurses: A continuation of the dialogue. *Nursing Forum, 3,* 53-56.

Heidgerken, L. R. (1973). Doctoral study in nursing. In *The doctorate in nursing science: A work conference,* (pp. 1-9). Washington, DC: School of Nursing, The Catholic University of America.

Holzemer, W. L. (1987, March/April). Doctoral education in nursing: An assessment of quality 1979-1984. *Nursing Research, 36*(2), 111-116.

Jamann, J. (Ed.). (1985). Proceedings of doctoral programs in nursing: Consensus for quality. *Journal of Professional Nursing, 1,* 90-100.

Kemble, E. (1966). Doctoral preparation for nurses: A continuation of the dialogue. *Nursing Forum, 3,* 39-44.

Lambertson, E. C. (1976). Projecting doctoral manpower requirements in nursing: A look at the criteria. In T. P. Phillips (Ed.), *Conference on doctoral manpower in nursing.* (DHEW Publication No. (HRA) 76-18. p. 73–79). Bethesda, MD: U. S. Department of Health, Education and Welfare, Public Health Service, Division of Nursing.

Lancaster, L. E. (1985). A comparison and development of models for the Doctor of Philosophy in Nursing and the Doctor of Nursing Science Degree. (Doctoral dissertation, Vanderbilt University, 1982). Ann Arbor: University Microfilm International.

Lash, A. A. (1987). Rival conceptions in doctoral education in nursing and their outcomes: An update. *Journal Nursing Education, 26*(6), 221–227.

Leininger, M. (1976a). Doctoral programs for nurses: A survey of trends, issues, and projected developments. In T. P. Phillips (Ed.), *The doctorally prepared nurse. Report of two conferences on the demand for and education of nurses with doctoral degrees.* (DHEW Publication No. (HRA) 76-18). Bethesda, MD: U. S. Department of Health, Education and Welfare.

Leininger, M. (1976b, May/June). Doctoral programs for nurses: Trends, questions, and projected plans. Trends, questions and issues on doctoral programs. Part 1. *Nursing Research, 25,* 201–203. Part 2. *Nursing Research, 25,* 204–210.

Matarazzo, J. D., & Abdellah, F. G. (1971, September/October). Doctoral education for nurses in the United States. *Nursing Research, 20,* 404–414.

McManus, L. (1960, October). Doctoral education in nursing: A nurse educator responds. *Nursing Outlook, 8,* 543–546.

Murphy, J. F. (1981). Doctoral education in, of, and for nursing: An historical analysis. *Nursing Outlook, 29*(11), 645–649.

Murphy, J. F. (1984). Essential resources for developing a doctoral program in nursing. *Nursing Educator, 9*(4), 6–10.

Murphy, J. F. (1985). Doctoral education of nurses: Historical development, programs and graduates. *Annual Review of Nursing Research, 3,* 171–189.

Nahm, H. (1966). Doctoral preparation for nurses: A continuation of the dialogue. *Nursing Forum, 5*(3), 36–39.

National League for Nursing. (1987). *Doctoral programs in nursing: 1986–1987.* New York: National League for Nursing.

Peplau, H. E. (1966). Nursing's two routes to doctoral degrees. *Nursing Forum, 5*(2), 57–67.

Rogers, M. E. (1966). Doctoral education in nursing. *Nursing Forum, 5*(2), 75–82.

Schlotfeldt, R. (1966). Doctoral study in basic disciplines—A choice for nurses. *Nursing Forum, 5*(2), 68–74.

Shores, L. S. (1986). Opening a doctoral program in nursing: Factors to consider. *Nursing Outlook, 34*(6), 286–288.

Snyder-Halpern, R. (1986). Doctoral programs in nursing: An examination of curriculum similarities and differences. *Journal Nursing Education, 25*(9), 358–365.

Taylor, S. D., Gifford, A. J., & Vian, J. (1971, September/October). Nurses with earned doctoral degrees. *Nursing Research, 20,* 415–427.

Tschudin, M. S. (1966). Doctoral preparation in other disciplines with a minor in nursing. *Nursing Forum, 5*(2), 50–56.

3

The Race for Resources: Who Can, Who Does, and Who Should Obtain Them?

Bonnie L. Rickelman, EdD, RN
Billye J. Brown, EdD, RN, FAAN

In the evolution of professional nursing, the number of doctoral programs is proliferating at a rapid pace. This situation creates a challenge to deans and faculties to amass the human and material resources necessary to ensure the continued existence and excellence of their doctoral programs. The competition for human and material resources among the diverse doctoral nursing programs raises the questions: Who can, who does, and who should obtain the available resources? This chapter addresses these questions within the framework of the indicators of quality for doctoral programs, including the criterion areas of faculty, programs of study, students, resources, research, and program evaluation (American Association of Colleges of Nursing, 1987), and considers several related problems and issues. These additional problems and issues include the acceleration of doctoral nursing programs, the focus of doctoral nursing curricula, enrollment profiles, society's need for doctorally prepared nurses, and types of resources that are currently available and needed in the future to support doctoral nursing education.

We acknowledge that the profile of doctoral program quality is multidimensional and that there is no precise definition of quality in graduate education (Pelczar, 1985). Nevertheless, since it is likely that doctoral nursing programs that meet the specified indicators of quality will have a competitive edge over those which only partially meet such standards, it seems pertinent to utilize the indicators of quality framework to organize this discussion and its basic question of who *should* obtain the resources for doctoral nursing education.

INDICATORS OF QUALITY IN DOCTORAL
NURSING PROGRAMS

There are a growing number of studies and opinions regarding indicators of quality in doctoral programs in nursing (Holzemer, 1982; American Association of Colleges of Nursing, 1985; Chioni, 1985; Holzemer & Chambers, 1986; American Association of Colleges of Nursing, 1987). In 1984 the Division of Nursing, Department of Health and Human Services, and the American Association of Colleges of Nursing (AACN), concerned about the present and the future of doctoral education, cosponsored an invitational conference on "Doctoral Programs in Nursing: Consensus for Quality" (Jamann, 1985). The purposes of the conference were to reach consensus on issues of quality in doctoral programs in nursing, to define critical areas needing quality control, to establish criteria for assessing quality, and to identify resources and extra-university relationships crucial to the operation of such programs. In 1986 the AACN membership endorsed the indicators of quality in nursing recommended by the 1984 conference. These indicators, or standards, complement those specified by the Council of Graduate Schools in the criterion areas mentioned previously, i.e., faculty, programs of study, students, resources, research, and program evaluation (AACN, 1987).

FACULTY

Quality indicators identified for the criterion, faculty, refer to doctorally prepared faculty members who hold graduate school appointments (if appropriate) in the university, are actively involved in research related to doctoral students' programs of study, disseminate new knowledge via publication of research and scholarly activities, and serve as mentors to students (AACN, 1987). Holzemer and Chambers (1986) state that the most significant standard for assessing the quality of a doctoral program is the scholarship of the faculty, including quality and quantity of publications, the amount of intramural and external funding secured, academic rank, and participation in professional activities. However, it has been noted that within schools of nursing, the commitment of the faculty to research productivity continues to be influenced by academic responsibilities which are more complex than those of most of our colleagues in nonclinical disciplines (Hinshaw & Sorensen, 1986; Brodie, 1986). The comparatively few doctorally prepared faculty members are struggling to balance responsibilities in the domains of teaching (often in both graduate and undergraduate clinical areas), university committee responsibilities, supervision of dissertations and theses, community service, student advising, consultation activities, and grant writing and research.

Brodie (1986) has observed that the increased involvement in the grant writing and research process by the faculty of doctoral programs has resulted in both positive and negative impacts on nursing education. Positive results include an increase in the prestige of nursing education within the state and nation, and consequently an increased ability to attract highly qualified persons as faculty members and students to the scholarly community. On the negative side, the increased pressure on faculty members to engage in research often results in their perceiving other essential business of the institution, such as developing courses, teaching, and serving on committees, as unproductive and not worthy of merit recognition. Thus, while a doctoral program may bring benefits to an institution, it may also divert funds and faculty members from other university commitments. A critical question that remains to be answered is: "What should be the relationship between research and the other dimensions of a professional career in a doctoral nursing program?" (Brodie, 1986, p. 350)

Brodie (1986) states that "the undergraduate program, especially during the last decade of financial stringency, has borne the heaviest burden in the shift in emphasis from teaching to research," and that "in research oriented universities, undergraduate teaching is viewed as neither interesting nor desirable, and . . . to be avoided by serious researchers at the peril of their careers" (p. 352). However, as the number of doctorally prepared faculty increases, it is likely that they will teach in undergraduate programs and that their activities in research and publishing will continue. A key question is: "How will the quality of the undergraduate program be assured as faculty increase their research and scholarly activity?" (p. 350).

It is unfortunate that such issues and problems have grown out of doctoral nursing education and the increased emphasis on research. However, they must be confronted and resolved if baccalaureate, master's, and doctoral nursing programs are to stay viable without leading to first and second class faculty and student status. All of these programs are currently essential to meeting society's needs for nursing practitioners, educators, administrators, consultants, scholars, and researchers who can positively influence health care and at the same time advance the knowledge base in nursing science. Can schools of nursing which offer the baccalaureate, master's, and doctoral programs ensure quality for each? Schools that succeed in this endeavor would surely deserve first consideration for supporting resources.

It is generally recognized that there is a link between a research oriented faculty and the receipt of various research moneys which can benefit the entire institution. Therefore, as for the questions of who can, who does, and who should obtain these funds, it seems pertinent to consider that success in building and maintaining a scientific community within a faculty helps ensure further receipt of moneys. Hinshaw and Sorensen (1986) discuss the process of developing a research oriented faculty and the types of resources available for this task. These authors point out that during the 1970s grants were available for faculty and research development, and schools of nursing that received these grants were thus provided a firm foundation for the next phase of research facilitation, the encouragement of faculty members to design research projects and to obtain moneys to implement investigations.

The two most important factors identified by Hinshaw and Sorensen (1986) as vital to the establishment and growth of a scientific community at The University of Arizona were the development of the doctoral program and the receipt of a Nursing Research Emphasis (NRE) grant. Other schools of nursing have validated the importance of such factors in building and maintaining a scientific community. Schools which have received NRE grants have promoted research by their faculties and have provided doctoral students with the opportunity for employment as research assistants on various projects. Thus there appears to be an evolutionary process for developing research productivity among faculties in schools of nursing. It involves obtaining research development resources, establishing a visible research structure within the school (such as a center for nursing research), and decisions by faculty members to view themselves as researchers and scholars and to conduct research relevant to the doctoral programs of study within their institutions (Hinshaw & Sorensen, 1986).

Faculty Credentials

In a national survey, 259 representatives from schools of nursing were asked to estimate their need for doctorally prepared faculty (Anderson, Roth, & Palmer, 1985). Responses indicated that doctorally prepared faculty were desired for 78 percent of the total budgeted positions, however, due to the unavailability of faculty members with doctorates, 42 percent of these positions were filled by non-doctorally prepared faculty. The investigators concluded that those nursing school faculty members who hold tenure-track positions but do not hold the doctoral degree must be encouraged to attain doctoral preparation. If they do not, it is likely that an already strained cadre of doctorally prepared nursing faculty will experience unreasonable workload demands in teaching, research, and scholarly endeavors, and in supervising theses and dissertations.

On the brighter side, it appears that the percentage of faculty members with doctoral degrees is increasing. In 1974 the number of full-time, doctorally prepared faculty members teaching in baccalaureate and higher degree programs was reported to be 621, while in 1986, this number was reported to be 2,176 (National League for Nursing, 1988a). Of the full-time faculty in baccalaureate programs, 23.7 percent hold doctorates, while 60.6 percent of the faculty who teach in both undergraduate and graduate programs hold doctorates. Of the faculty teaching only at the graduate level, 63.5 percent have a doctoral degree (NLN, 1988a).

PROGRAMS OF STUDY

According to AACN (1987), quality indicators for doctoral programs include both core and cognate content; nursing history and philosophy related to the development of nursing knowledge; existing substantive nursing knowledge; theory construction and research methodologies; data management, tools, and technology; and social, ethical, and political issues in nursing. In addition, high quality doctoral programs maintain clearly written program requirements that are available to students, and their faculties are responsible for determining the program of study and methods of instruction. However, there are challenges which the nursing profession must confront in its efforts to establish and maintain quality doctoral programs which compete for supporting resources: 1) the proliferation of doctoral programs in nursing, and 2) the substantive focus of doctoral curricula.

Proliferation of Doctoral Programs in Nursing

In 1960, there were only 4 doctoral programs in nursing. This increased to 30 by 1984, and by 1989 48 institutions offered 50 doctoral nursing programs. Of these, 34 offered the PhD only, 1 offered both the PhD and the DNS, 1 offered both the PhD and DNSc, 1 offered the DSN, 4 offered the DNS, 6 offered the DNSc, and 1 offered the EdD (American Association of Colleges of Nursing, 1988a; University of North Carolina, personal communication, May, 1988). Table 1 presents these doctoral programs in nursing by institution and type of degree. It had been predicted that there could be as many as 70 doctoral nursing programs in the United States by 1988 (AACN, 1985). This number had not been reached at the beginning of 1988; however, another prediction of 65 doctoral programs by 1995 may hit the mark (Brodie, 1986).

While the growth in the number of doctoral nursing programs must continue, it should come in an orderly progression which balances the educational needs of the profession with available societal resources. The decision to initiate a doctoral nursing program should be based on societal need as demonstrated by local, regional, and national surveys; evidence of qualified potential students; evidence of potential for a high quality program (including secure funding; adequate library, computer, and laboratory facilities; and qualified faculty who have a demonstrated record of scholarly productivity, service, and high quality teaching in undergraduate and graduate nursing). Careful deliberation must be given to the decision to open new doctoral nursing programs that might merely duplicate existing programs as well as exacerbate the competition for students, faculty, and scarce financial resources. Once the need for new doctoral programs has been clearly established and resources have been identified, sites for the programs and the types of degrees to be offered can be selected.

However, determining society's needs for doctorally prepared nurses and designing the curricula to meet those needs are tasks currently made difficult by such related problems as declining enrollments in baccalaureate schools of nursing, decreased funding and public support for nursing education, and the expanded opportunities for women in other career fields (Shaw, 1987). To ensure the continued viability of doctoral programs in

TABLE 1.　Doctoral programs in nursing by
institution and type of degree (N = 46)*

Institution	Degree	Institution	Degree
Adelphi Univ (NY)	PhD	Univ of Colorado	PhD
Boston Col (MA)	PhD	Univ of Florida	PhD
Boston Univ (MA)	DNSc	Univ of Illinois	PhD
Case Western Reserve		Univ of Iowa	PhD
Univ (OH)	PhD	Univ of Kansas	PhD
Catholic Univ (DC)	DNSc	Univ of Kentucky	PhD
Columbia Univ,		Univ of Maryland	PhD
Teachers' College (NY)	EdD	Univ of Miami (FL)	PhD
George Mason Univ (VA)	DNSc	Univ of Michigan	PhD
Georgia State Univ/		Univ of Minnesota	PhD
Medical Col of Georgia	PhD	Univ of North Carolina	
Indiana Univ	DNS	—Chapel Hill	PhD**
Louisiana State Univ	DNS	Univ of Pennsylvania	PhD &
Loyola University of Chicago	PhD		DNSc
Med. Col of Virginia—		Univ of Pittsburgh (PA)	PhD
Va Commonwealth Univ	PhD	Univ of Rhode Island	PhD
New York Univ	PhD	Univ of Rochester (NY)	PhD
Ohio State Univ	PhD	Univ of San Diego (CA)	DNS
Oregon Health Sciences Univ	PhD	Univ of South Carolina	
Rush Univ (IL)	DNSc	—Columbia	PhD
State Univ of New York		Univ of Tennessee	
(SUNY)—Buffalo	DNS	—Memphis and Knoxville	PhD***
Texas Women's Univ	PhD	Univ of Texas at Austin	PhD
Univ of Alabama		Univ of Utah	PhD
—Birmingham	DSN	Univ of Virginia	PhD
Univ of Arizona	PhD	Univ of Washington	PhD
Univ of California,		Univ of Wisconsin—Madison	PhD
Los Angeles	DNSc	Univ of Wisconsin—Milwaukee	PhD
Univ of California		Wayne State Univ (MI)	PhD
—San Francisco	PhD & DNS	Widener Univ (PA)	DNSc

*Note. Data from AACN (1988), Newsletter, 14(1), 3.
**Note. Data from personal communication, May, 1988.
***Note. Data from personal communication, February, 1989.

nursing, Shaw (1987) suggests that administrators and faculty members utilize a proactive marketing plan based on Hunt's (1983) "Proactive Marketing Model" to attract students to nursing programs. This proactive plan involves assessing the school's market—for doctoral education in this case—including community and societal needs for doctorally prepared nurses, characteristics of the university's program, characteristics of existing competitors, and potential students (Shaw, 1987).

It is not known how many doctoral nursing programs have systematically used such a marketing plan to assess the needs of society for doctorally prepared nurses and to plan their doctoral programs to meet the needs identified. However, in a study to analyze deans' perspectives on decisions to initiate doctoral programs in nursing, Shores (1986) asked whether a feasibility study was used during the decision-making process. She found that only 2 out of 25 schools had conducted such a study. Moreover, 37 percent of the schools reported surveying higher education coordinating bodies, but none had surveyed state legislatures. Sixty-eight percent of the schools responding indicated that the prevention of program duplication was important regionally, but 63 percent responded that the prevention of program duplication at the state level was not applicable for their state. Forty-one percent of the respondents indicated that a computer facility was the only one needed for the initiation of a doctoral program. Only 51 percent of the respondents indicated that hiring additional faculty would be necessary in their particular schools, but 100 percent of the respondents thought that an adequately prepared faculty is essential (Shores, 1986). It would be interesting to know whether these perspectives would hold true were this study replicated in the current context of doctoral program proliferation. Since states usually limit the money they spend on higher education, it would seem prudent to include state legislatures in feasibility surveys.

Why are the numbers of new doctoral programs in nursing burgeoning? Are new doctoral programs being established primarily for the purpose of bringing funds into the school? If so, what will happen to the doctoral programs when funding dwindles? When the federal government provided funds for graduate psychiatric nursing education during the 1960s and 1970s, the number of nurses choosing to obtain their advanced degrees in this specialty area increased. However, when the money was withdrawn, enrollment in those graduate nursing programs declined. Will we see a repeat of this phenomenon in other areas of doctoral nursing preparation?

Other generally repeated perspectives on why doctoral nursing programs are increasing are that research will not be produced in a school lacking a doctoral program; or the belief that the only way to recruit doctorally prepared faculty is to have a doctoral program; or the fear of losing external research funding unless a doctoral program is in place. Are any of these perceptions accurate? The mission of the parent organization determines whether research is to be included among the activities of its faculty. However, there is no reason to suppose that those individuals in schools and colleges which do not include research as a part of their mission could not be engaged in research. In fact, information which appears later in this chapter from the National Center for Nursing Research (NCNR) of the National Institutes of Health, the Division of Nursing, Sigma Theta Tau International, and the American Nurses' Foundation, refutes the contention that a nursing school must have a doctoral program in place to obtain research funding. Those programs that do obtain research funding should be those that meet established indicators of quality in research.

Doctoral Curricula in Nursing

At a conference sponsored by the AACN in February 1988, entitled "Doctoral Preparation for the Future: Planning Now to Meet the Need," a key question was asked which may influence the receipt of funding resources and which demands the attention of the nursing profession. It asks: "What should be the focus and substantive content in doctoral programs in nursing?" (American Association of Colleges of Nursing, 1988b).

In a related discussion of form versus substance in doctoral education, form courses were identified as research methodology courses, theory courses, and process courses; and substantive courses were identified as content focused. Is the focus of doctoral nursing education to be simply methodological? Dr. Shaké Ketefian, a participant at the AACN conference, noted that some faculty members are in a "research cocoon," doing their own particular research and teaching research and theory courses. Ketefian questioned whether they ever emerge to teach essential content courses in the doctoral program. Further exploration of the fit between form and substantive content courses in nursing doctoral programs seems necessary. Those doctoral programs in nursing which educate primarily for research and theory development methodology at the expense of substantive knowledge in a clinical content area may find that their graduates are viewed by society as not being clinically knowledgeable or as not making beneficial contributions to consumer health care. It is clear that there must be a balanced integration of research and theory development methodology with substantive clinically oriented content in doctoral programs, and research investigations relevant to patient care needs and health promotion.

STUDENTS

Indicators of doctoral program quality for the criterion, students, include the following: a pool of qualified applicants; admission criteria consistent with those of the parent institution; a clearly defined financial assistance program for doctoral students who have equal opportunity to compete with doctoral students in other disciplines for university-sponsored financial assistance; academic advising; and continuity of assistance from the faculty to achieve research objectives (AACN, 1987). The federal government has been the strongest source of financial support for nurses enrolled in doctoral programs. In a 1979-1980 survey of 1,964 doctorally prepared nurses, Brimmer, Skoner, Pender, Williams, Fleming, and Werley (1983) found that 44 percent of their respondents reported federal support for their doctoral education; 40 percent reported support from government grants, and 4 percent reported having received government loans. The next most frequently reported sources of financial support were university fellowships and assistantships (18%). However, 16.4 percent of the respondents indicated that they had received no financial support for their doctoral studies during the years 1975-1979, possibly reflecting a downturn in the federal government's support for health education during that period.

It is essential that faculty members serving as graduate advisors and/or academic advisors be familiar with the various financial assistance programs at their respective institutions and encourage their qualified students to apply for these competitive awards along with doctoral students from other disciplines. With increasing enrollments in doctoral nursing programs, there will be strong competition for both intra- and extramural financial assistance for students.

Enrollment Profiles

The number of enrollments in doctoral nursing programs was reported at 1,949 in 1986, a 220 percent increase from 1976 and a 9 percent increase from 1985 to 1986 (NLN, 1988b). After a gradual decline in full-time enrollments since 1980, there now appears to be a slight increase in full-time enrollments. Geographic profiles of enrollees in doctoral nursing programs indicate that the North Atlantic and South have the largest groups of enrolled doctoral students, with about 31 percent each. Enrollments in the Midwest comprise 22 percent, while the West reports 1.6 percent of the total doctoral student enrollment.

In 1975–1976, only 59 students graduated from doctoral nursing programs, while in 1985–1986, 249 students graduated, representing a 322 percent increase over this 10-year period (NLN, 1988b). The largest number of doctoral graduates occurred in the South, with over 31 percent of the total, followed by the North Atlantic with 30, the Midwest with 21, and the West with 18 percent, respectively.

While it is hoped that many baccalaureate and master's degree nursing graduates will choose to obtain doctoral degrees in nursing, it is particularly disturbing that from 1976–1986, baccalaureate enrollments declined 19 percent, including a 10.3 percent decline from 1985 to 1986. Enrollments in master's programs have increased only 2.6 percent from 1984 to 1985 and only 3.3 percent from 1985 to 1986, indicating a stabilization in these enrollments (National League for Nursing, 1988b). Perhaps these data reflect the prediction that, from 1979 to 1994, the numbers of students in the 18–24 year old age group would decrease by approximately 25 percent (Keller, 1983). If so, nursing, along with other disciplines, will have to recruit students from other markets, resulting in a shift in student clientele, especially at the baccalaureate and master's levels. Economic restraints and job retrenchments in some disciplines, along with an increasing awareness of the current nationwide nursing shortage, are propelling students with baccalaureate degrees in disciplines other than nursing to seek admission to nursing schools. Some nursing programs have had the foresight to plan and implement innovative programs, such as the master's as the first professional nursing degree, for these alternate career students. Graduates of such programs then become potential student resources for doctoral programs.

Regarding the question of which programs should obtain resources to support doctoral education, it would seem that this may be judged in part by the quality of the students admitted to the various doctoral programs, and their contributions as graduates in advancing the nursing profession and the health care of society. Students seek a quality of doctoral education that prepares them with the most recent knowledge and with marketable skills for positions in demand by society. What are society's views regarding the need for doctorally prepared nurses?

Need for Doctorally Prepared Nurses

In 1984 there were approximately 1.5 million nurses in the United States. Of these, about 4,900 or 0.3 percent were prepared at the doctoral level, and were employed as follows: faculty positions in academic settings and in clinical inservice, 2,952 (60.2%); administrators or assistant administrators, 1,151 (23.5%); consultants, 207 (4.2%); staff nurses, 369 (7.5%); clinical nurse specialists, 137 (2.8%); and other, 85 (1.7%) (U.S. Department of Health and Human Services, 1984).

During the mid-1980s, Anderson and associates (1985) surveyed 169 health service agencies nationally to determine the estimated need for doctorally prepared nurses. The respondents represented a fairly even distribution between public and private agencies, including home health agencies, academic health centers, health departments, medical centers, magnet hospitals, and military nursing services. These respondents were asked to identify the projected need for doctorally prepared nurses within the next five years (1983-1988).

Of the 71 home health agencies, 37 (52%) identified a need for one or more doctorally prepared staff members, with the areas of greatest need being ranked as 1) doctoral preparation in administration, and 2) doctoral preparation with a strong clinical focus. Seventy-two respondents represented academic health centers. Their estimated need for doctorally prepared nurses ranged from 0-30, and, like the respondents from the home health agencies, they expressed the greatest need for nurses with administrative expertise followed by nurses with clinical specialist doctoral preparation.

Of the 29 respondents from public health departments, 13 (45%) did not prefer doctorally prepared nurses in job positions, while 15 (52%) preferred to have between 1 and 3. One large health department indicated a desire for doctorally prepared nurses in 25 of the available positions. Unlike the home health agencies and the academic health centers, the health departments desiring doctorally prepared staff indicated their greatest need was for those prepared as clinical specialists rather than as administrators. When asked how many positions for doctorally prepared nurses were desired by magnet hospitals, 7 of the 21 respondents (33%) reported none, 10 (48%) reported between 1 and 4, and 4 (19%) reported needing between 5 and 9 positions. Chiefs of Nurse Corps respondents from the Army, Navy, and Air Force, and Directors of Nursing in V.A. hospitals all indicated an increased need for doctorally prepared nurses in clinical positions within the next 5 years.

Several questions arise from the findings of this survey concerning both the felt need for doctorally prepared nurses and the type of doctoral preparation desired. What was the basis for the response by some of the agencies that they did not want any doctorally prepared nurses in the immediate future? Are the numbers and types of budgeted positions for nurses a limitation in recruiting those who are doctorally prepared? Have there not been sufficient numbers of doctorally prepared nurses in such positions to document their value, or for the agencies to make an informed judgment as to their need? Or perhaps, are the positions in these agencies of such a nature that the highest quality of service is achieved by individuals with less educational preparation?

It is noteworthy that the findings from this survey show agreement between schools of nursing (findings discussed earlier) and most health agency respondents that clinical practice expertise is often the most highly desired area of preparation for both doctorally prepared faculty and those nurses working in various health service agencies. Insofar as these findings reflect the opinions and identified needs of similar agencies and institutions, it would seem that those doctoral programs which emphasize substantial clinical knowledge and research skills meet society's demand for such graduates, and consequently should rank high in terms of receiving available resources for program support.

RESOURCES AND RESEARCH

Since there is an increased emphasis on nursing research throughout all sectors of the nursing profession, the quality indicators for the criteria of resources and research will be examined together. The measures of quality for the criterion, resources, as related to doctoral programs have been identified as adequate computer, library, clinical and laboratory facilities, and financial and institutional means to support both program and student needs (AACN, 1987). Similarly, quality indicators for the criterion, research, include adequate facilities and funding to support research by the faculty and the dissemination of research findings through publications and presentations to learned societies; faculty research congruent with the school of nursing's program goals; and student research congruent with the faculty's research strengths. In addition, the institution's research goals should emphasize solving clinical problems and validating clinical nursing interventions (AACN, 1987).

Roncoli, Brooten, and Perez-Woods (1988) note that the research process is expensive in terms of both direct and indirect costs and they wonder whether nurses and nursing are willing to meet these costs. Although no dollar figures are mentioned, direct costs are identified as outlays for such items as "equipment, laboratory tests, printing questionnaires, paper, photocopying, pens and pencils, postage, telephone charges, computer time and supplies, secretarial support, consultant fees, research assistant fees, and other personal costs," including the percentage of the researchers' salaries while they are doing the research (Roncoli, et al., 1988, p. 77). While small grants may be obtained from many universities to help ease these costs, it is usually necessary to seek external funding. The biggest indirect cost of research is the "release time" which most investigators must negotiate from their institutions in order to develop and implement a research proposal. Other indirect costs include space for consultation meetings and storing materials, analyzing data, and writing and disseminating the study results (Roncoli, et al., 1988).

In 1985, the Cabinet on Nursing Research of the American Nurses' Association (ANA) issued a document entitled "Directions for Nursing Research: Toward the Twenty-First Century." Goals outlined in this document include an increase in the number of nurse-scientists by the year 2000; the generation of knowledge regarding the optimum functioning and wellness of individuals; excellence in nursing education; the development of clinical and academic environments supportive of nursing inquiry; and the dissemination of nursing research results to the public and health care policy makers. If such goals are to be reached, additional funding, both public and private, will be needed for the research of nursing school faculty members and clinicians, and for expanded support for pre- and postdoctoral training, new investigators, and mid-career development awards (Cabinet on Nursing Research, 1985).

Funding Resources

An exploration of all the available funding resources is beyond the scope of this chapter. However, a discussion of research priorities and types of funding to support doctoral program needs as outlined by the National Center for Nursing Research, the Division of Nursing, Sigma Theta Tau International, and the American Nurses' Foundation follows.

National Center for Nursing Research

Within the National Center for Nursing Research (NCNR), the Division of Extramural Programs (DEP) oversees three areas of research programs: 1) Health Promotion/Disease Prevention, 2) Acute and Chronic Illness, and 3) Nursing Systems. On the basis of a survey of general and specialty organizations in nursing, the NCNR has identified seven priority areas in which it will consider grant applications for research in nursing (Hinshaw, 1988, June). These seven priority areas will give researchers some direction about what types of research projects are appropriate to future grant applications. They are:

1. Bio-psycho-social components of care for HIV positive clients and their partners and families

2. Care of low birth weight infants and their families, with a focus on prevention of complications and innovative nursing care delivery patterns

3. Quality of care for long-term conditions, including a focus on nursing home care, patient and caregiver coping and adaptation, and continuity of care

4. Clinical assessment and symptom management for acute illness phenomena

5. Informational systems, including development of a taxonomy of nursing care phenomena and standardized data sets which document nursing care across settings

6. Health promotion parameters, with emphasis on lifestyles, self-care, and the development of health promoting behaviors among adults and children

7. Technological dependency across the lifespan, with a focus on individual and family responses and prevention of iatrogenic complications

At its February 1988 meeting, the NCNR National Advisory Council approved proceeding with priorities 1 and 2 as named above and were scheduled to further consider the other priorities at a June 1988 meeting (Hinshaw, 1988, June).

In fiscal year (FY) 1987, the total budget for the NCNR was $20 million. In FY 1988, the budget was $23,380,000, and the projected President's budget for FY 1989 is $31.5 million (Hinshaw, personal communication, June 6, 1988). According to Hinshaw, only a portion of the NCNR budget is used to fund those projects dealing with identified priorities. The remaining part is used to fund meaningful and creative individual research endeavors (Hinshaw, 1988, June). The amount of moneys allocated to each type of research was not specified. The NCNR will continue to establish its research programs "as independent of, but complementary to, the research activities supported by other components of the NIH" (National Center for Nursing Research, 1988a, p. 6). In addition, investigators are encouraged to establish their own nursing research programs and to participate in collaborative research with researchers from other institutions that receive funds from the various NIH Institutes. Currently, the NCNR is preparing a document regarding "Research Career Trajectory," which will discuss the stages and essential components of research career development for postdoctoral, midcareer, and senior level nurse researchers (Hinshaw, 1988).

NCNR Grant Mechanisms of Support. Currently, 13 types of grants are awarded to institutions by the NCNR on behalf of a principal investigator (National Center for Nursing Research, 1988b):

1. **Traditional Research Project Grant (R01):** Supports (up to 5 years) specific projects related to an investigator's interests and competence. Researchers are encouraged to complement ongoing activities and to utilize existing resources in NIH-supported centers.

2. **Academic Research Enhancement Award (AREA) (R15):** Supports feasibility studies and small scale research projects by faculty members in educational institutions which have not been major participants in NIH programs. Eligibility is limited to US baccalaureate and higher degree programs in the sciences related to health. Awards can be for up to $35,000 per year for 3 years.

3. **First Independent Research Support and Transition Award (FIRST) (R29):** Supports first independent investigative efforts of an individual with the goal of effecting a transition toward traditional

types of NIH research projects. Awards are for 5 years, not to exceed $350,000 and researchers must commit at least 50 percent of their time to the project in each budget period.

4. **Method to Extend Research in Time (MERIT) (R37):** Provides continuing long-term support for excellent and established investigators who have already received a 5-year grant. Awards are made for R01 applications.

5. **Program Project Grant (P01):** Supports a broadly based, often multidisciplinary, research program with a specific major objective or theme. Individual investigators conduct discrete research projects related to the overall program objective.

6. **Academic Investigator Award—Nursing (AIA) (K07):** Provides support up to a maximum of $60,000 in direct costs for salary and fringe benefits for 3 to 5 years for junior faculty members who are 4 to 6 years beyond their doctorate. Awardees must commit at least 75 percent of their time to conducting the research.

7. **Clinical Investigator Award—Nursing (CIA) (K08):** Provisions are similar to those of the AIA; awards are made to doctorally prepared, clinically trained nurses to encourage development into independent investigators. Awardees must work under a sponsor at an NIH-supported Center program or in a General Clinical Research Center (GCRC) funded by the Division of Research Resources (DRR) of the NIH.

8. **Cooperative Agreements (U01):** This grant involves greater participation of the NCNR staff in project planning and decision making than does a traditional or regular research grant. Applications are solicited by the NCNR or other NIH Institute.

9. **Institutional National Research Service Award (NRSA) (T32):** Provides support for eligible US institutions that have the required program director, faculty, and facilities to provide pertinent predoctoral and/or postdoctoral research training for nurses. Grant funds are primarily for trainee stipends. Trainees are selected by the institution.

10. **Individual NRSA Predoctoral Fellowship (F31):** Provides support for supervised research training leading to a doctoral degree in areas related to the mission of the NCNR. Applicants must be registered nurses with either a baccalaureate or a master's degree in nursing.

11. **Individual NRSA Postdoctoral Fellowship (F32):** Provides support for postdoctoral training related to the NCNR mission for registered nurses or non-nurses holding a doctoral degree.

12. **NRSA Senior Fellowship (F33):** Provides support for nurse investigators who hold a doctoral degree and have had at least 7

subsequent years of relevant research or professional experience at the time of the award. Allows investigators to take time from regular professional responsibilities to increase capabilities for implementing research.

13. **Small Business Innovation Research Award (SBIR) (R43/R44):** Provides grants to small businesses with the technological expertise to contribute to NIH's research and development mission.

As of March 1, 1988, the NCNR listed 145 active research awards. Most of these awards are for direct clinical nursing intervention studies and for the study of health related behavioral phenomena. Regarding the question of who does obtain research moneys, the schools of nursing which received 3 or more of these research awards (amounts not specified) during this time period are as follows (NCNR, 1988b):

University	No. of Awards
The University of Washington	13
University of Michigan (Ann Arbor)	10
University of Colorado (HSC)	7
The University of California (SF)	6
University of Maryland (Baltimore)	6
Oregon Health Sciences Center	5
University of Arizona	5
University of Illinois	4
Case Western Reserve	4
University of Nebraska Medical Center	4
University of Wisconsin—Madison	4
University of Iowa	3
The University of Texas at Austin	3
University of Rochester	3
University of North Carolina, Chapel Hill	3
City of Hope Medical Center (California)	3
Ohio State University	3

The Division of Nursing

Additional financial resources to support both master's and doctoral nursing education are available from the Bureau of Health Professions, Division of Nursing, US Department of Health and Human Services, in the form of: 1) Professional Nurse Traineeships (PNT), 2) Special Project Grants, and 3) Advanced Nurse Education Grants. The PNTs are awarded to currently licensed professional nurses through grants to public or private nonprofit educational institutions providing master's and doctoral degree programs whose graduates will serve as nurse practitioners, nurse administrators, nurse educators, nurse researchers, or other nursing specialists. Public or private nonprofit schools of nursing and other institutions which educate nurses as nurse midwives also may be awarded PNTs. The PNTs provide for tuition, fees, and stipends up to

$6,552 per year for a maximum of 36 months of study. Since fiscal year 1964, approximately $283.3 million has been made available for this program. In 1986, 171 grants were funded for about $11 million, assisting an estimated 4,320 students (Division of Nursing, Bureau of Health Professions, 1987a). Applications are mailed annually to eligible institutions.

The Special Project Grants aim "to improve nursing practice through projects that increase the knowledge and skills of nursing personnel and enhance their effectiveness in care delivery" (Division of Nursing, Bureau of Health Professions, 1987b). Examples of special projects include:

1. Assisting individuals from disadvantaged backgrounds to obtain nursing education, and providing counseling or pre-entry education designed to facilitate their successful completion of the regular course of nursing education

2. Providing continuing education for nurses

3. Providing pertinent retraining opportunities for nurses who desire re-entry into active nursing

4. Demonstration projects related to improved geriatric training in preventive care, acute care, and long-term care, including home health care and institutional care

5. Increasing the supply of specialty nursing personnel required to meet the health needs of the nation

6. Providing training to upgrade the skills of licensed vocational or practical nurses, nursing assistants, and other paraprofessional nursing personnel

7. Demonstration projects related to clinical nurse education programs which combine educational curricula and clinical practice in acute-care facilities, long-term care facilities, and ambulatory-care facilities

8. Demonstration projects to improve access to nursing services in noninstitutional settings, such as nursing practice arrangements in communities

9. Demonstration projects to encourage nursing graduates to practice in areas of health manpower shortage

Since fiscal year 1965, $268.5 million has been available for the Special Projects program. In 1986, 73 grants and contracts were funded for about $10.3 million (Division of Nursing, Bureau of Health Professions, 1987b).

Regarding the Advanced Nurse Education Grants, these grants are awarded "to assist eligible institutions to increase the number of registered nurses prepared as nurse educators, administrators, researchers and nursing specialists" (Division of Nursing, Bureau of Health Professions, 1987c). Public and nonprofit collegiate schools of nursing are eligible to apply for support to implement advanced nurse education projects designed to 1) plan, develop, and operate; 2) expand; or 3) maintain programs at the master's or higher level to prepare nurses as indicated above. Since the initiation of this program in 1975, about $129 million has been made available to schools of nursing. In fiscal year 1986, 107 awards were made totaling $15.6 million.

Sigma Theta Tau International

Sigma Theta Tau International has provided research funding since 1936. When this organization's research fund was established in 1934, the stated purpose of the fund was "to foster development of scientific attitude in relation to nursing problems, to give financial aid in the execution of research in this field, to help awaken nurses to the fact that there is need for research in nursing" (Sigma Theta Tau International, 1934, p. 1). The early amounts of these research awards ranged from $50 to $500, depending on the nature of the problem and the expenses involved. The awards were available to any nurse who demonstrated an ability to implement research and whose study was viewed as benefiting the nursing profession (Sigma Theta Tau International, 1934). The focus of the research funded by Sigma Theta Tau has ranged from infant development to experiences of the aged; from the effects of chemotherapy to the management of hypertension and study of various psychiatric variables (Westwick, 1980). Since 1936, Sigma Theta Tau has awarded 173 grants totaling $343,795, with an average of $1,987 per scholar (N. Watts, Executive Officer, Sigma Theta Tau International, personal communication, May 26, 1988).

A summary of the educational levels of grant recipients during the years of 1976–1987 reflected the following educational levels (reported by percentage): doctorate (49%); doctoral candidate (36%); master's (14%). During this period, the grant requirements included the master's degree as the minimum criterion for application. In 1987, 9 grants were awarded for a total of $37,075, with an average award of $4,119. From 1976 to 1987, approximately 27 percent of the grants submitted were funded.

In 1988, out of 70 grant applications, 16 (23%) were recommended for funding. The educational levels of the grant recipients were as follows: doctorate (87.5%); doctoral candidate (6.25%); and master's (6.25%) (N. Watts, personal communication, May 26, 1988).

The American Nurses' Foundation

The American Nurses' Foundation (ANF) has provided funds for research since 1955. Since then, over 300 nurse scholars have received approximately $1.2 million in competitive extramural grants (ANF, 1988). Early awards were given for such study topics as the work of the general duty nurse and the private duty nurse; registered nurses in metropolitan communities; patterns of psychiatric nursing; and the nurse–patient relationship in the healing process. More recently, however, the focus of the studies which have received awards is more clinically oriented, focusing on such clinical phenomena as care of hypertension, osteoarthritic women, pulmonary artery pressures, factors in pain alleviation and other care related topics. Additional topics have included the homeless, historical phenomena, and various organizational problems.

In 1987, 27 nursing research grants were awarded for an average of $2,600 per scholar. Although these grants may be awarded to non-nurses, more nurses than non-nurses have received them. The grants are awarded to individuals with baccalaureate, master's, and/or doctoral degrees.

Of the 327 grants awarded from 1955 to 1987, 5(1%) were awarded to individuals with baccalaureate degrees; 115 (35%) went to master's prepared individuals; 198 (61%) were awarded to doctorally prepared individuals; and 10 (3%) went to individuals whose educational credentials were unknown (American Nurses' Foundation, 1988). Of the colleges or universities receiving ANF grants, approximately 48 percent currently have doctoral programs in nursing, indicating that ANF moneys have been awarded to institutions which do not have doctoral programs. However, of the 46 doctoral programs in nursing, approximately 84 percent have received ANF grants (ANF, 1988). In 1987, a new collaborative grant was initiated, entitled "The American Nurses' Foundation/Sigma Theta Tau International Scholar Award." This grant is available in the amount of $6,000 to a master's prepared scholar for research on a clinically oriented topic, with the review of the proposal based on its scientific merit (N.E. McCormick, American Nurses' Foundation, personal communication, June 3, 1988).

Although funding sources from both public and private sectors continue to support nursing education, practice, and research, financial support for research in all fields usually falls short of needs and expectations (Infante, 1987). In the face of massive budget deficits at the federal level, there may be future cuts in funding for nursing programs and projects (McKibbin, 1983). Thus, the race for resources among institutions with doctoral nursing programs will continue to be keenly competitive. Those institutions that use strategic planning and evaluation methods to ensure program quality will likely be the ones to stay in the race.

EVALUATION OF PROGRAM

Specified quality indicators for doctoral program evaluation include those parameters previously discussed, i.e., the knowledge which the program contributes to nursing; the accomplishments of students, faculty, and alumni; faculty and student qualifications; policies and operational procedures; the learning environment; intra- and extramural resources; and the quality of student, faculty, and alumni research (AACN, 1987). Who rates the quality of institutions and their doctoral programs? National surveys have been used to assess quality in doctoral programs as early as the 1920s (Pelczar, 1985). Although specific national surveys are not discussed here, readers are referred to Pelczar (1985), Chamings (1984), and Gourman (1985) for information regarding such surveys. National surveys have commonly evaluated quality in relation to the ranking and reputation of the institutions and their programs and research-related activities. Generally, the respondents in such surveys are deans, department chairpersons, and faculty members. However, it should be noted that the ranking of institutions and their graduate programs via national surveys has received a fair share of criticism. The raters may be biased and the "halo effect" rather than objective information may influence high rating of programs at elite institutions; the surveys often do not contribute knowledge useful to improving programs; large institutions may receive high ratings for emphasis on research and scholarship at the expense of teaching and undergraduate education; survey results may be misused; and a single set of criteria may not determine the quality of all programs, since the objectives of graduate programs differ (Pelczar, 1985).

Nevertheless, the issue of quality must continue to be confronted by administrators, faculty members, and alumni of doctoral nursing programs. Most schools of nursing have strategic planning and evaluation processes to assess the quality of life of their programs in place. The degree to which these programs excel in the specified areas of quality is likely to determine who can, who does, and who should obtain the resources to support doctoral nursing education and research.

SUMMARY

Several impressions result from the information presented in this chapter. First, in order to maintain a population of potential doctoral nursing students, schools of nursing which have both undergraduate and graduate programs must avoid operating these programs in isolation, or attempting to emphasize the meaningfulness of one over the other. Since knowledge generated at the graduate level usually filters down to applicable utilization at the undergraduate level, graduate and undergraduate research-oriented faculty should participate willingly in teaching and socializing undergraduate nursing students to become capable consumers of research and users of research findings in practice decisions. Second, those nursing programs with continuing track records for generating meaningful research and producing graduates who compete well in the marketplace and who make positive contributions to society and to the profession will likely obtain the resources they need to remain viable. Such programs will continue to attract research-oriented faculty and moneys to support research and programs. However, administrators and faculty members in doctoral nursing programs must be concerned about whether the public views the nursing practice, research, and theory development efforts of these programs as beneficial to the public's nursing needs and health care. Thus, there is a need for academic nursing to inform the public about the accomplishments of its faculty, students, and alumni and the associated benefits which accrue to society.

Third, with the increased number of doctoral programs and graduates, we may soon experience a glut of doctorally prepared nurses. During the ensuing hiatus of student enrollment, there may be a need for more innovative uses of graduate faculties and graduate students, during the course of which doctoral programs will work even harder at marketing themselves to ensure their survival and continued excellence.

Finally, as Brodie (1986) observes, ". . . the same set of historical circumstances do not repeat themselves in the same configuration" (p. 353). Therefore, perspectives and answers regarding the questions of who can, who does, and who should obtain the resources to support doctoral nursing education will continue to be determined as the profiles of society's health care needs change and influence nursing education, practice, and research.

REFERENCES

American Association of Colleges of Nursing. (1985). *Proceedings of Doctoral Programs in Nursing: Consensus for Quality.* Meeting held August 13-15, 1984. Cosponsored by the American Association of Colleges of Nursing and the Division of Nursing, Department of Health and Human Services, Washington, DC.

American Association of Colleges of Nursing. (1987). Position statement: Indicators of quality in doctoral programs in nursing. *Journal of Professional Nursing, 3*(1), 72-74.

American Association of Colleges of Nursing. (1988a). Doctoral preparation for the future: Planning now to meet the need. Conference held February 22-24, 1988, San Antonio, TX.

American Association of Colleges of Nursing. (1988b). *Newsletter.* Washington, DC, *14*(1), 3.

American Nurses' Foundation, Inc. (1988). *Competitive extramural grants program: Awards (1955-1987).* Kansas City, MO.

Anderson, E., Roth, P., & Palmer, I. S. (1985). A national survey of the need for doctorally prepared nurses in academic settings and health service agencies. *Journal of Professional Nursing, 1*(1), 23-33.

Brimmer, P. F., Skoner, M. M., Pender, N. J., Williams, C. A., Fleming, J. W., & Werley, H. H. (1983). Nurses with doctoral degrees: Education and employment characteristics. *Research in Nursing and Health, 6,* 157-165.

Brodie, B. (1986). Impact of doctoral programs on nursing education. *Journal of Professional Nursing,* November-December, 350-357.

Cabinet on Nursing Research. (1985). *Directions for nursing research: Toward the twenty-first century.* Kansas City, MO: American Nurses' Association.

Chamings, P. A. (1984). Ranking the nursing schools. *Nursing Outlook, 32*(5), 238-239.

Chioni, R. M. (1985). Discussion: Areas in which quality control is essential. *Journal of Professional Nursing, 1*(2), 108-109.

Department of Health and Human Services. (1984). *The registered nurse population*, November (HRP-0906938). Washington, DC: U.S. Department of Commerce, National Technical Information Service.

Division of Nursing. (1987a, February). *Fact sheet: Professional nurse traineeships*. Washington, DC: Bureau of Health Professions, U.S. Department of Health and Human Services.

Division of Nursing. (1987b, February). *Fact sheet: Special project grants*. Washington, DC: Bureau of Health Professions, U.S. Department of Health and Human Services.

Division of Nursing. (1987c, February). *Fact sheet: Advanced nurse education grants*. Washington, DC: Bureau of Health Professions, U.S. Department of Health and Human Services.

Gourman, J. (1985). *The Gourman report: A rating of graduate and professional programs in American and international universities*. Los Angeles: National Educational Standards.

Hinshaw, A. S. (1988, June). *Proud to care about nursing research: National Center for Nursing Research*. Paper presented at the American Nurses' Association Convention, Louisville, KY.

Hinshaw, A. S. (1988). The National Center for Nursing Research: Challenges and initiatives. *Nursing Outlook, 36*(2), 54–56.

Hinshaw, A. S., & Sorensen, G. E. (1986). Researchmanship: The University of Arizona—Productivity versus resources. *Western Journal of Nursing Research, 8*(2), 243–247.

Holzemer, W. L. (1982). Quality in graduate nursing education. *Nursing and Health Care, 3*(11), 171–189.

Holzemer, W. L., & Chambers, D. B. (1986). Healthy nursing doctoral programs: Relationship between perceptions of the academic environment and productivity of faculty and alumni. *Research in Nursing and Health, 9,* 299–307.

Hunt, S. D. (1983). General theories and the fundamental explanation of marketing. *Journal of Marketing, 47*(3), 9–17.

Infante, M. S. (1987). Nursing educational research: planning to achieve our future. *Patterns in Nursing: Strategic Planning for Nursing Education* (pp. 107–116). New York: National League for Nursing.

Jamann, J. S. (Ed.). (1985). *Proceedings of Doctoral Programs in Nursing: Consensus for Quality*. Sponsored by the American Association of Colleges of Nursing and the Division of Nursing, Department of Health and Human Services, August 13–15, 1984. *Journal of Professional Nursing, 1*(2), 90–121.

Keller, G. (1983). *Academic strategy: The management revolution in American higher education*. Baltimore: The Johns Hopkins University Press.

McKibbin, R. C. (1983). Nursing education trends: An analysis of the supply and preparation of nursing personnel. *Education for nursing practice in the context of the 1980s.* Kansas City, MO: American Nurses' Association.

National Center for Nursing Research. (1988a). *Nursing science: Serving health through research,* April 4, 1988. (Available from NCNR, National Institutes of Health, Building 38A, Room B2E17, Bethesda, MD, 20894.)

National Center for Nursing Research. (1988b). *Report of active research awards as of 3-1-88.* (Available from NCNR, National Institutes of Health, Building 38A, Room B2E17, Bethesda, MD, 20894.)

National League for Nursing. (1988a). *Nursing data review 1987.* New York: National League for Nursing, Division of Research.

National League for Nursing. (1988b). *Nursing student census with policy implications.* New York: National League for Nursing, Division of Research.

Pelczar, M. J. (1985). The nature of the doctorate and criteria for quality. *Proceedings of Doctoral Programs in Nursing: Consensus for Quality.* Sponsored by the American Association of Colleges of Nursing and the Division of Nursing, Department of Health and Human Services, August 13–15, 1984. *Journal of Professional Nursing, 1*(2), 94–100.

Roncoli, M., Brooten, D., & Perez-Woods, R. (1988). Nursing research: What it costs and who will pay. *Nursing and Health Care, 9*(2), 77–80.

Shaw, R. J. (1987). Proactive marketing in nursing education. *Nurse Educator, 12*(5), 11–15.

Shores, L. S. (1986). Analysis of decisions to initiate doctoral programs in nursing. *Nurse Educator, 11*(1), 26–30.

Sigma Theta Tau International. (1934). *Research fund report,* 1.

Westwick, C. (1980, May-June). *Reflections.* 2.

4

Achieving Program Approval: The Proposal and the Process

Patricia R. Forni, PhD, RN, FAAN

INTRODUCTION

The development and approval of a doctoral program is clearly a long, tedious process. Initial planning to final approval may involve a decade or more of proposal development, submission, revision, and resubmission. This chapter explores the elements of the proposal development and approval process as described by 32 doctoral programs in nursing, and based upon personal experience of the author in program development and a review of the literature.

SURVEY OF DOCTORAL PROGRAMS

Survey Sample

Current information was compiled by a survey conducted during the spring/summer of 1988. A questionnaire was mailed to the directors of 34 recently developed doctoral programs in nursing who replied with a 94 percent (N = 32) response rate. Of these 32 programs, 22 percent (N = 7) had been approved in the 1970s and the remainder in the 1980s. Data from all respondents were used in the analysis. Eight respondents also provided copies of proposals and one submitted a copy of a needs assessment.

Findings

The year of program approval as reported by survey respondents may be found in Table 1. Since 1985, 18 new programs have received approval. This represents 39 percent of the existing programs at the time of this writing (N = 46).

TABLE 1. Year of program approval
for selected doctoral programs.

Year Approved		Number
1971		1
1974		1
1975		2
1977		1
1978		2
1981		1
1982		2
1983		2
1984		2
1985		7
1986		7
1987		2
1988		2
	Total	32

The regional representation of responding programs by type of control is in Table 2. The greatest number of new programs were represented in the South with 12 programs having been developed, 11 of which were in public institutions. The greatest number of privately controlled programs were represented in the East where 5 programs were developed. Twenty-four (75%) of the 32 responding programs were located in public institutions.

By far the greatest number of programs offered the PhD, with 25 (78%) out of 32 programs offering this degree. The remaining programs offered the DNS or DSN; none offered both degrees.

Programs reported a time span of 0 to 17 years for program approval from date of initial proposal submission to final approval. These data are found in Table 3. By far the greatest number of programs (N = 28) were approved within 2 years from date of submission.

Program directors were asked in what year and how many students were admitted. Most respondents reported having admitted students either in the same year or within one year of receiving approval. The range in number of students admitted was 1 to 33. All but 1 program admitted 10 or fewer students. The initial enrollment modes were 5 or 10 students with 5 programs each reporting these enrollments. A total of 21 programs (65%) initially enrolled between 5 and 10 students. These data are reported in Tables 4 and 5.

The majority of programs (N = 21 or 65%) reported approval upon first submission. Programs reporting they were not approved upon first submission were asked what components of the proposal were addressed in the recycle. Three programs reported that the need for the program required further elaboration. Other factors mentioned were program content, learning activities and behaviors, student enrollment and progression, workload and faculty recruitment, qualifying exams, financial resources, and political negotiations. No consistent theme was noted among programs needing to resubmit.

TABLE 2.   Location of program by region and
type of control for selected doctoral programs.

Location	TYPE OF CONTROL	
	Public	Private
Midwest		
Illinois		1
Iowa	1	
Kansas	1	
Michigan	1	
Minnesota	1	
Ohio	1	
Wisconsin	2	
Subtotal	7	1
South		
Alabama	1	
Florida	1	1
Georgia	2	
Kentucky	1	
Louisiana	1	
North Carolina	1	
South Carolina	1	
Tennessee	1	
Texas	1	
Virginia	2	
Subtotal	12	1
West		
Arizona	1	
California	1	1
Oregon	1	
Utah	1	
Subtotal	4	1
East		
Massachusetts		1
New York	1	2
Pennsylvania		2
Rhode Island	1	
Subtotal	2	5
Total	25	8

A feasibility study was conducted by 27 out of 31 reporting programs. The study was required of 18 programs primarily by a statewide system or board of regents. Other reported sources for requests were the graduate school, the provost, the faculty, a program evaluator, or the study was required by a federally funded grant.

Programs were asked what components were addressed in the proposal. Each one addressed the following components: the need for the program, feasibility study results (among those who conducted one), faculty qualifications/ productivity, and resources of the institution/school. Other responses to the

TABLE 3.   Time span from
proposal submission to approval
for selected doctoral programs.

Year(s)	Number
Unknown	1
0	4
½	1
1	15
1½	1
2	7
3	1
10	1
17	1
Total	32

components may be found in Table 6. It is readily apparent that, of the other components, faculty resources, secretarial support, assistantships for students, library, equipment, and space were the most frequently cited elements that were included in the proposal. Reported under the "other" category were research support, five-year plan, computer facilities, funding, comparison with programs in like institutions, and competition with existing non-nursing doctoral programs.

Student financial aid was addressed by 21 programs (one respondent replied "don't know"). The most frequently mentioned type of aid was assistantships. Also mentioned were scholarships and federal nurse traineeships.

Federal funding from the Division of Nursing, DHHS, was obtained by 16 programs (50%) with an additional 1 pending and 1 disapproved. Only two other sources of external funding were cited and both were from private foundations. Of those reporting funding, amounts cited ranged from $162,000 to $1,395,465 over a three-year period. The latter amount was from 3 separate grants.

Respondents were asked to describe characteristics of the proposal that strengthened its passage; 27 programs responded. Documentation of need was the most frequently cited response (N = 10). Faculty productivity and

TABLE 4.   Interval between approval and admission
of doctoral students for selected doctoral programs.

Interval (years)	Number	Percent
Admitted same year	12	38
One	17	53
Two	2	6
Three	1	3
Total	32	100

TABLE 5. Number of doctoral students initially
admitted for selected doctoral programs.

Number of Students	Number	Percent
1	1	3
2	1	3
3	3	9
4	3	9
5	5	16
6	3	9
7	2	6
8	3	9
9	3	9
10	5	16
33	1	3
Unknown	2	6
Total	32	

qualifications, especially in research, also were cited as being important. Other characteristics mentioned were: curriculum design, use of visiting professorships, quality of the proposal in terms of completeness and clarity, strength of master's program, being the first nursing doctoral program in state, the feasibility study results, letters of endorsement, the fact that no additional resources were requested, the pool of potential applicants, support from nursing community, political homework, internships, intensive personal lobbying, and compatibility with university goals.

Programs were asked to identify factors that weakened the passage of the proposal. There was no clearcut theme in these responses, however, evidence indicated that nursing was not regarded as a scholarly discipline and this was viewed as presenting a distinct weakness. Several programs mentioned problems due to lack of understanding of nursing science, nursing theory, and the PhD in

TABLE 6. Selected components addressed in
the proposal for selected doctoral programs.

Component	Number	Percent
Faculty	31	97
Secretarial staff	24	75
Assistantships	22	70
Student workers	10	31
Library	28	87
Travel	16	50
Commodities (supplies)	3	9
Equipment	25	78
Telephone	13	41
Space	24	75
Other	7	22

TABLE 7.   Source of letters of endorsement
for selected doctoral programs.

Source	Number	Percent
University colleagues	24	75
Nursing leaders	25	78
Community at large	14	44
Other	7	22

nursing. There were problems cited due to multiple nursing programs within the state(s) seeking approval at the same time, as well as factors of limited funded research by faculty, program costs, length of program, and political resistance.

Twenty-three or 71 percent of the programs employed consultants either for program development, for the feasibility study, or as part of the review process. Ten programs indicated that use of consultant(s) was required; most often the state higher education body or board of regents requested it. In a few cases consultation was asked for by the graduate school. All programs reported the consultants to be helpful.

Of those programs responding (N = 30), only two reported that they did not request letters of endorsement. The remaining programs obtained letters from university colleagues, nursing leaders, and the community at large. These data are reported in Table 7. Other sources of endorsement mentioned were university administration, visiting committee, prospective employers, clinical agencies, the state governor, consumers, and representatives of other state system universities.

Summary

Eighteen or 39 percent of the existing doctoral programs in nursing were developed in the past 3 years (1985–1988) according to this 1988 survey, with the greatest number of programs in the responding sample being in the South (N = 12). Most programs were in public institutions (N = 24 or 75%). The PhD was the most frequently offered degree (N = 25). It took as long as 17 years to achieve program approval (N = 1) but the mode was 1 year (N = 15). Most programs (N = 29) admitted students within a year following approval and all but 1 program admitted 10 or fewer students initially. It is interesting to note that the majority of programs (N = 21 or 66%) reported approval upon first submission. Among programs resubmitting their proposals, there was no theme noted regarding areas that were addressed in the recycle. Most programs conducted feasibility studies (N = 27) while it was required of only 18. Important elements of the proposal which were frequently addressed were need for the program, feasibility study results, faculty qualifications/productivity, resources of the school/institution, and student financial aid. Many programs (N = 16) received federal funding from the Division of Nursing, DHHS. Programs cited convincing statements of need as the most important characteristic of the proposal for strengthening its passage. Some programs reported that the view of nursing as not being a scholarly discipline was a distinct weakness. Most programs employed consultants (N = 23) and obtained letters of endorsement (N = 28).

THE PROPOSAL

Long years of planning are involved in the development of a doctoral program in nursing. Although no step-by-step procedure can be prescribed, there are essential elements that must be addressed.

Planning

Part of the planning process includes assessment of the school's/institution's readiness to offer a doctoral program. The American Association of Colleges of Nursing's (AACN) *Position statement: Indicators of quality in doctoral programs in nursing* (1985) provides an excellent source of indicators for gauging a school's readiness along the six parameters identified: faculty, programs of study, resources, students, research, and evaluation of program.

Faculty, according to the indicators, should be actively engaged in research relevant to the program of study and to the phenomena of nursing; should have graduate school appointments; hold earned doctorates; publish in refereed sources; serve as mentors for socializing students; be accessible; and participate in the community of scholars.

Programs of study, according to the indicators, should contain certain common elements of content: history and philosophy; nursing knowledge; theory construction; social, ethical, and political issues; research design and method; data management; and student research opportunities. There should be provision for core content and cognates; faculty should determine the curriculum and how it will be taught; and written policies and procedures should be available.

Resources, according to the indicators, should include computer services; library; appropriate laboratories; clinical research centers (if applicable); clinical facilities; and financial and institutional resources.

Indicators relative to **students** include a qualified student pool; rigorous admission criteria with opportunity for review of "exceptional" applicants who do not meet the criteria; availability of program information and career counseling; encouragement of all students to enroll full time; activities for professional socialization; continuity of faculty assistance with research; adequacy of resources and services; a financial assistance program and opportunity and encouragement to participate in funding competition.

Research indicators include adequate research funding from the school and university; research facilitating activities for faculty; research role expectations of faculty; support for student research; expectations for presentation and publication of scholarly work; research that contributes to the body of nursing knowledge, supports program goals and includes clinical investigation; and postdoctoral training.

Program evaluation, according to the indicators, should address curriculum; students, faculty, and alumni including their accomplishments and/or qualifications; policies and procedures; the learning environment; contributions to nursing knowledge; resources and relationships; and quality of research (AACN, 1985).

In meeting the quality indicators, a school may decide it needs to strengthen its faculty complement in terms of research productivity, external funding of research activities, or faculty credentials in the disciplinary focus of the program (e.g., nursing administration, gerontology) or type of degree to be offered. Space may need to be acquired or renovated. Dialogue with other disciplines on campus may need to be initiated to enlist their support and to encourage the development of appropriate cognate courses. Computer resources may need to be upgraded. All of the above activities require considerable lead time, planning, and cultivation, not to mention the financial means that may be required to accomplish them.

Need/Justification

The establishment of a need for the program is an essential component in the development process. This factor was mentioned by survey respondents more frequently than any other as the one lending strength to the proposal. The feasibility study can be used to provide original data in support of need. National, regional, and state data sources also are helpful. Two important sources of data supporting the need are the reports of the Institute of Medicine (1983) and the Western Interstate Commission for Higher Education (1978). The latter document provides estimates of need within lower and upper boundaries and both national and state estimates are given. In addition to these sources, some states have developed statewide planning documents for nursing and data from these sources that may be of assistance. An excellent source of data on regional need is *Planning for doctoral nursing education in the South* (McPheeters, 1985).

Need versus demand may become an issue which needs elaboration. The above cited sources of need data (IOM and WICHE) are based upon estimates of job opportunities for individuals with these qualifications to provide services in health care, education, consultation, administration, and research. McPheeters (1985, p. 50) states that, "the need is the number that experts judge to be required; the demand is the number who are actually employed or enrolled." He further differentiates two dimensions as the, " . . . (1) need and demand of the marketplace for doctorally prepared nurses, and (2) the need and demand of nurses for doctoral education in nursing."

Demonstration of need in the job market surely lends support to development of a doctoral program. Employment opportunities can be demonstrated through feasibility study data obtained in surveys of potential employers. It is important to have data from a variety of job settings including both educational and service sectors. Demonstrating that employment opportunities are available in educational settings is relatively easy, but it is more difficult to support their availability in service settings. It is helpful to have letters of support from potential employers attesting to their need and interest in employing doctorally prepared nurses.

Letters of support from colleagues in other nursing programs, service settings, and other disciplines also lend credibility to the need.

Purpose/Objectives. Often the proposal format requires that the program purpose and objectives be included. Whether required or not, this is an important element to consider, as it gives form and meaning to the program's structure and academic base. It may be helpful as well to relate the program purpose to the overall purpose/mission of the institution.

Background Information. Because doctoral education in nursing is a relatively recent phenomenon it may be helpful to include some historical data about development of doctoral education in nursing in the United States as well as some explanation of the discipline of nursing. The latter presentation may provide a means of addressing some of the difficulties reported earlier.

Duplication of Effort. In every proposal it will be necessary to address existing programs in the area (usually the state) that are similar to the one being proposed. If duplication will exist, a strong case must be made as to why the proposed program is needed and how it will be different from existing programs in the area. This is especially important for programs proposed for states or perhaps regions where doctoral nursing programs already exist. The case may be made that the proposed program will differ in (1) degree offered (DNS or PhD); (2) curriculum focus/content; (3) location and demographics of applicant pool; (4) program costs (public supported programs are usually less expensive); and (5) accessibility of resources.

Program Fit with School/Institutional Resources. Another component of the justification has to do with program fit within the institutional mission/goals. This often includes statements about the service region, student clientele, programmatic goals, research goals, and institutional/school of nursing resources. Consideration should be given to whether the resources of the school and the institution are of sufficient quantity and quality to support the proposed program. This consideration applies to all elements of the proposal. If a research-based doctorate is being proposed, the following questions need to be addressed: Are there nursing faculty in sufficient numbers who are actively engaged in externally funded research? Are there sufficient doctoral level cognate courses in other disciplines to support the minor and the research/statistical components of the program? If a practice-based doctorate is being proposed: Are there nursing faculty in sufficient numbers who are engaged in the application of research in the clinical settings? Are there sufficient clinical facilities to provide for student research and practice?

Are there sufficient doctoral level cognate courses in other disciplines to support the functional role?

Faculty

Factors related to the faculty which deserve attention include the following:

Qualifications and Productivity. The most important program components contributing to the success of the proposal are the qualifications and productivity of the faculty. Is there a community of scholars contributing to the development of the knowledge base in nursing? The answer to this can be provided in the evidence of scholarly productivity among the faculty who will be participating in the proposed doctoral program. Evidence includes information concerning funded faculty research (source and amount), publications, consultations, research presentations, editorial board memberships, peer reviews for grants, and other evidence of national reputation as judged by one's peers. Evidence of expertise and ongoing experience in the designated nursing specialty of the proposed program also is vital if the practice-based degree is being proposed. Experience in serving on dissertation committees, either in nursing or in other disciplines, is another factor that is valued by those reviewing the proposed programs. Information about faculty qualifications and productivity should be included in the appendices.

A critical mass of faculty with credentials in the discipline must be available to teach in the program. This means that if the PhD is to be offered there must be faculty with PhDs in nursing to teach in the program; if the DNS is to be offered the same principle applies. This is not to say that faculty with doctorates in other disciplines or faculty with other doctoral degrees (DrPH or EdD for example) cannot lend expertise to the proposed program. Early on in the development of doctoral programs in nursing, it was both necessary and sufficient to utilize faculty with non-nursing doctorates. This practice parallels the early development of master's programs in nursing when faculty with non-nursing master's degrees were utilized. However, the cadre of nurses with doctorates in the discipline is growing and should be tapped for employment in these new programs.

Faculty Size. The number of faculty needed for the proposed doctoral program depends on program size and content and allocation of credit for dissertation advisement, faculty research, or other special requirements. If additional faculty are required, plans for their recruitment should be addressed. According to McPheeters (1985, p. 11), "Each program requires a critical mass of seven such faculty persons."

Program Requirements

Program requirements which need to be further addressed include:

Curriculum. The proposal will include a narrative description of the proposed curriculum, course descriptions, and sample program progressions. Some rationale may be necessary to explain how or why the program is developed or organized the way it is. Some explanation also may be required as to the relationship of the proposed doctoral curriculum to the master's level curriculum. This is certainly indicated if modifications need to be made in the master's curriculum.

Admission. Admission requirements of the nursing program and of the graduate school, if the program comes under the purview of the latter unit, must be described.

Tool Requirements. Tool requirements include specific skill development, such as languages, statistics, theory development, or computer applications, that are necessary for the program. These requirements should be described and a rationale presented, as related to the proposed curriculum as a whole and the nature of the degree.

Other Special Requirements. Requirements for residence, assistantships, the program advisory committee, the qualifying committee and examination, the comprehensive examination, the dissertation committee, and defense must be included in the proposal. The sequencing of these events for progress in the program should also be stated. Both policies and procedures for implementing them must be developed and may or may not be required as a part of the proposal.

Cognate Courses. The availability of cognate or supporting courses to be offered by other disciplines should be addressed. A list of these courses provided in an appendix may be helpful to reviewers as well as letters of support from cooperating departments.

Evaluation. Some proposal formats call for a statement describing how the proposed program will be evaluated.

Resources

Support resource requirements also need elaboration in the proposal in terms of:

Space. The proposal must address how the proposed program will be accommodated in the way of space. Will existing space within the unit be reallocated? Will new space be required? Will renovation of space be necessary? If so, at what expense and in what timeframe? Will additional faculty have to be accommodated? Will additional space be necessary for graduate assistant offices, study areas, seminar and conference rooms, support staff, computer facilities, laboratories, research, etc.?

Library. Library resources should be detailed in terms of existing resources and those necessary to implement and sustain the proposed program. Availability of inter-library and consortial arrangements should be described. Special library features such as access to computer searches may be mentioned. The institution's library staff may assist in preparing this section of the proposal.

Support Staff. The way in which the proposed program will be supported in terms of secretarial/clerical or other support staff assistance should be addressed. Will existing personnel absorb the doctoral work or will new personnel be required? If new personnel are to be added, consideration must be given to where they will be housed and to the furniture and equipment they will need.

Computer Facilities. A description of access to computers and computer laboratories is an essential part of the program proposal. Facilities of both the school of nursing and the university should be described including their availability to doctoral students and faculty. Plans for acquisition of additional hardware and software to support the proposed program need to be addressed.

Equipment. Should any special equipment be required it should be described in terms of both housing for it and source of financing.

Laboratory Facilities. Laboratory requirements for biomedical or behavioral research, laboratory animals, and laboratory equipment must be addressed in the proposal. Space and sources of funding for both the acquisition and maintenance must be included.

Clinical Facilities. Access to clinical facilities that will support program goals is essential and should be described in the proposal. If special clinical considerations are needed they should be described as well. Letters of support from participating clinical sites will be helpful.

Students

The proposal must address special features of the program that are concerned with the students.

Student Demand. Demonstration of student demand will be necessary. Data supporting student demand can be gained from either the feasibility study or published resources. Two relatively easy sources of potential student samples that can be tapped are the school's alumni and current enrollees in NLN accredited master's programs in nursing. The institutions to be surveyed can be identified in the current issue of the NLN's *Master's education in nursing: Route to opportunities in contemporary nursing*. Institutions selected for a survey can be initially queried as to their willingness to participate. If they agree, questionnaires can be sent to them for distribution to master's students.

Student demand data also can be generated from faculty who currently teach in baccalaureate and master's programs in nursing and who lack doctoral preparation. Another source is the nursing population in clinical settings; however, they are not as easy to access. Expressions of interest, intentions to enroll, and actual enrollments are quite different phenomena. Nevertheless, expressions of student interest and intent provide useful information for inclusion in the proposal. Some states have conducted statewide studies that address student demand for doctoral education. Illinois, for example, conducts a biennial survey of nursing personnel, in conjunction with license renewal, that is funded by dedicated money from the renewal fee. (State of Illinois, Department of Registration and Education, 1987).

Student Pool. Data regarding the potential applicant pool are more readily available from published sources. The annual members of baccalaureate and master's graduates are available from a variety of sources. The AACN publishes data on this periodically (AACN, 1988), and information is available from the American Nurses Association's *Facts about nursing 86–87* (1987).

Size of Program. As noted earlier initial enrollments of students tend to be small. All but one program in the previously reported survey had an enrollment of ten or fewer students initially. Student enrollment, of course, is determined by the resources of the institution; most importantly, the faculty resources to provide adequate guidance and supervision of the dissertation or clinical practicum or internship. McPheeters (1985, p. 10) reports that, "The 'typical' program that will be most cost beneficial has a class size of 15 students, a faculty of 8 full-time faculty, and costs of $18,450 per student per year," although 10 to 15 students is also cost beneficial but " . . . raises the average cost per student per year to $20,000 . . . ."

Student Financial Aid. Student financial aid is an important component of the proposal; doctoral education is both lengthy and expensive. Sources of financial aid, both institutional and external, should be identified. A new initiative from the Division of Nursing, DHHS, is the Post-baccalaureate Faculty Fellowship which provides tuition and fees and a monthly stipend for faculty engaged in the last year of dissertation work on specified subject areas. Funding for these fellowships is subject to continuing support from Congress.

Impact on Other Programs

The initiation of a doctoral program will require accommodation in the organizational structure of the academic unit as well as consideration of its impact on other programs. Change(s) in organizational structure usually are not addressed in the proposal. The impact of the proposed program on budget allocations, faculty qualifications and workload, and curricular requirements in the nursing master's programs are areas that may be discussed. The impact of the proposed program on the other academic units that will provide support courses also may need to be considered in terms of enrollment, need for course development, and budgetary items.

Program Funding

A significant part of the proposal deals with how the proposed program is to be funded. Will new resources be required? If so, for what specific items or categories? One school that responded to the survey had completely revamped its master's program curriculum in conjunction with development of the doctoral program. Significantly reducing the credit hours required at the master's level meant that the doctoral program could be implemented without additional state funds. Funding also may be sought from private foundations or federal sources.

Deciding whether to offer full-time or part-time enrollment is another consideration. Part-time enrollment is allowed in many programs. McPheeters (1985, pp. 60–61) says that, "While part-time arrangements are not the ideal pattern for doctoral education, the reality is that over half of the potential candidates for doctoral education in nursing cannot afford to take full-time doctoral work." Nonetheless, programs would be well advised to give serious consideration to the impact that part-time enrollment will have on program costs.

THE PROCESS

The Decision

The decision to undertake development of a doctoral program constitutes the initial major step in the process and must be made only after study of a substantial body of related and reliable evidence. Often, the assembly and analysis of this information represents such a significant outlay of time and resources that the nature of the decision may be unduly influenced by the effort. In any case, the decision may be made either by an individual or by a group or committee, but it eventually requires approval of the entire school faculty and ultimately of a variety of entities. Norris (1985) believes that the consequences of doctoral program development are far-reaching and may not be fully understood by faculties at the time of development. She projects a number of changes that will occur within five years after initiating a doctoral program. On the positive side there will be an upgraded faculty in terms of senior scholars and researchers, an improved research climate will exist, there will be more dynamic faculty-student relationships, nursing's position in academia will be strengthened, there will be growth in the theory and science of nursing as well in nursing methodology and instrumentation, individual program planning will be facilitated, and there will be improved communication among faculty (Norris, 1985). All of these changes must be accompanied by a faculty that is credentialled at the doctoral level and that is heavily committed to and involved in research and theory building/testing. Impact of the doctoral program on other school of nursing programs is not clearly understood, Norris maintains. She says faculty, " . . . do not foresee changes in faculty composition or modifications in the school budget" (Norris, 1985, p. 8) and as a consequence are likely to become angry and frustrated when these changes occur.

Someone or some entity must take responsibility for development of the proposal and guidance through the approval process. For the programs surveyed the most frequently mentioned source was a faculty committee, followed by a faculty member, the dean, and the associate/assistant dean. Obviously, program development is a group effort and it is important to enlist assistance early on.

Shores (1986) conducted a study in 1983 of 25 schools of nursing that had doctoral programs. One of the findings of her study was that, "A majority of the respondents believed that the presence of PhD programs in other disciplines on campus, medical center affiliation, and assessment of potential student and employer interest should be at least somewhat important to schools considering doctoral program initiation in the future" (p. 27).

Consultants

The utilization of consultants, whether mandatory or voluntary, is a popular practice among schools that have developed doctoral programs. Consultants may be brought in at various stages of program development or during the review process. It may be desirable to have different consultants for different parts of the process, for example, the school may wish to engage one consultant for assistance with curriculum early on and yet another for review of the proposal in general later. The graduate school, governing board, or the higher education board may require a consultant to assess the school's/institution's readiness to offer a doctoral program. The identity of the consultant may or may not be made known to the proposing program.

Feasibility Study

The feasibility study is really an assessment of various factors that support development of the doctoral program and give direction to that development. The factors include but are not limited to the following: whether there are potential students in sufficient numbers interested in enrolling in the proposed program; whether there are potential employers who would hire the graduates of such a program; what factors would contribute to the success of the program, such as special course scheduling (evenings, weekends, summers); need for student financial aid or housing; full-time or part-time enrollment preference; what the curriculum focus should be (research, specialty practice, administration, consultation, etc.); time preference for beginning the program; type of degree preferred; reason(s) for enrolling in a doctoral program; plan for financing doctoral education; and career goals.

Most institutions require that a feasibility study be carried out for new program approval. Questions to be addressed may be specified in institutional documents. Starck (1980), in describing the practical aspects of doing

a feasibility study, reminds us to first exhaust all existing data sources prior
to gathering our own data.

The Review/Approval Process

Internal. One cannot assume that approval of the doctoral program
proposal will sail through the nursing faculty. At this level of review/
approval, concerns tend to be of a different nature than those encountered
further along in the approval process. Faculty may feel threatened by the
prospect of a doctoral program for any number of reasons: they may lack
the terminal degree; their research, publications, and scholarly activities
may be lagging; or they may prefer the status quo and resist any change.
These are not insurmountable problems. Indeed several programs have reported that initiation of a doctoral program had a positive effect on the
entire ambience of the school. One of the consequences was that faculty
hurried to attain the terminal degree so that they could meet the requirements for teaching in the doctoral program.

Involvement of faculty from other disciplines in the development of the
doctoral program in nursing can facilitate its approval in the university gov-
ernance system. Appointment of an advisory committee with representation
from appropriate disciplines can pay off in several ways. It provides opportunity for (1) profiting from the expertise of the various disciplines represented;
(2) addressing any barriers/obstacles/objections prior to formal submission of
the proposal, and (3) gaining interdisciplinary support from the committee
members early on.

If the proposed program is the DNS or DSN, it may not be subject to the
scrutiny of the institution's graduate school, rather it may come under the
review of the graduate department of the nursing unit. This circumstance has
both advantages and disadvantages. While it may expedite the review process
by not having to undergo review by the graduate school, it also means that the
proposal will not necessarily have to meet the rigorous standards of that organizational unit.

The PhD program, being a research-based degree, does come under the
purview of the graduate school. As such, the proposal will be reviewed by the
interdisciplinary committees of that body. Having successfully gone through
this procedure the nursing school can be assured that the proposed program
meets the standards of the institution. It is probably at this level of review that
the proposal will go through its most serious, indepth test. The quality and
quantity of faculty research, grant funding, publications, and other scholarly
works will be closely reviewed and compared with the level of activity in the
other disciplines. Often nursing faculty are held to the same expectations for
funded research as faculty in the biomedical sciences where both opportunities and funding amounts are greater.

The graduate school may require that a consultant's report be part of the review process. In the survey described herein, three respondents reported that a consultant was required by the graduate school; four respondents reported that some statewide body required it; and five respondents reported that the institution's governing board required it.

Competition for scarce resources among schools within the institution may come into play at this level of review. This is especially true when there are other doctoral program proposals in the university for which financial support is required which are seeking approval in the same cycle.

Administrative Support. It is assumed that discussions with "higher administration" have taken place early in the planning process and there is agreement that the proposed program fits the institutional mission. Thus, by the time the proposal reaches the offices of the provost and the president, approval will be *pro forma*. The same case can be made regarding approval by the governing body of the institution.

External. Public-supported programs are subject to the review and approval of a statewide entity, such as a coordinating board or higher education board, that exercises control over the institution. Review at this level may be anything but *pro forma*. The proposal will be scrutinized for duplication of services if there are other nursing doctoral programs in the state or nearby in the region. Competition for resources at this level will be keen.

In at least one state, Illinois, there is a Commission of Scholars that is engaged by the Board of Higher Education to review and make recommendations regarding approval of all new doctoral programs in state-supported institutions. The Commission is comprised of scholars, representing various established disciplines, from prestigious institutions around the country. New doctoral programs are not approved without positive recommendation from the Commission.

Political Considerations

Political conditions vary from institution to institution and from state to state. No attempt will be made here to explore what those conditions might be or how to tackle them, except to say that this sensitive area cannot be ignored.

Another sensitive issue which will need to be addressed with considerable vigor, supported by factual and persuasive information, is the question of why nurses *need* doctoral education. There appear to be at least three possible reasons for this doubt: (1) a sexist orientation to nursing that it is a female dominated profession and that women do not need to be educated at that high a level; (2) a lack of understanding (or belief) that nursing has a body of knowledge all its own on which to base doctoral education; and (3) a lack of knowledge concerning the scope and value of nursing research. Coupled with this kind of thinking may be the belief that doctoral education, if attained, does not need to be in the discipline of nursing.

Luck

The role of luck in science, as in life, cannot be ignored. It also comes into play under many circumstances. The following incident is reported by Dr. Constance Baker* regarding the approval of the doctoral program at the University of South Carolina—Columbia, College of Nursing, while she was dean there. On the day the proposal was being presented to the Governor's Committee of the State of South Carolina, a step preceding the Commission on Higher Education review, the New York Times published a sizable news item extolling the research of one of the College of Nursing faculty. The major portion of the article by Jane Bryant, science editor, describing the scientific basis for nursing practice, was devoted to the federally funded research of the nurse faculty member.

When the Commission meeting opened, a statement was made reminding Dean Baker that the purpose of the PhD was to prepare scholars for a life of science, and asking her what research existed in the College of Nursing to support a PhD in nursing science. At that point, Dean Baker produced a copy of the New York Times with its bold headline describing the nursing research. Needless to say, this event had a very salutary effect on the presentation.

CONCLUSION

In some ways, the process may represent the most important factor since commitment to the development of a doctoral program is required throughout the process. Those involved need to hold strong beliefs regarding the value of doctoral education, must be learned about doctoral education, and must be able to articulate clearly their values and knowledge. The process itself is a vital learning experience for those who create the proposal.

A multitude of factors come into play in the development of a doctoral program proposal and its subsequent movement through the review/approval process. Not the least of these is the hard work required of the principal authors of the proposal. While politics and luck both play a role in the process and may be completely beyond the control of the nursing school or even the university, care in preparing and documenting the proposal are certainly indispensable.

There has been enormous growth in the number of doctoral nursing programs developed in recent years, but that growth appears to be tapering off. As programs continue to be developed, it will become increasingly important to address the parameters of the proposal and the process as outlined in this chapter.

*Recounted by permission of Dr. Constance Baker, currently dean at Indiana University, School of Nursing.

REFERENCES

American Association of Colleges of Nursing. (1985). *Position statement: Indictors of quality in doctoral programs in nursing.* Washington, DC: Author.

American Association of Colleges of Nursing. (1987). *Report on nursing faculty salaries in colleges and universities.* Washington, DC: Author.

American Association of Colleges of Nursing. (1988). *Report on enrollment and graduations in baccalaureate and graduate programs in nursing.* Washington, DC: Author.

American Nurses Association. (1987). *Facts about nursing 86–87.* Kansas City, MO: Author.

Institute of Medicine. (1983). *Nursing and nursing education: Public policies and private actions.* Washington, DC: National Academy Press.

McPheeters, H. L. (1985). *Planning for doctoral nursing education in the South.* Atlanta: Southern Regional Education Board.

National League for Nursing. (1987). *Master's education in nursing: Route to opportunities in contemporary nursing.* New York: Author.

Norris, C. M. (1985). The PhD in nursing program: A five-year projection. *Nurse Educator, 10*(2), 6–11.

Shores, L. S. (1986). Analysis of decisions to initiate doctoral programs in nursing. *Nurse Educator, 11*(1), 26–30.

Starck, P. L. (1980). Practical aspects of conducting a feasibility study for graduate education in nursing. *Journal of Nursing Education, 19*(4), 33–38.

State of Illinois, Department of Registration and Education. (1987). *1986 biennial survey of Illinois registered nurses.* Springfield, IL: Author.

Western Interstate Commission for Higher Education. (1978). *Analysis and planning for improved distribution of nursing personnel and services.* Hyattsville, MD: U. S. Department of Health, Education and Welfare.

5

Doctoral Faculty as a Community of Scholars: Positive Environments for Doctoral Programs

Elizabeth R. Lenz, PhD, RN

The doctorate is the degree of scholarship. Regardless of the type of degree awarded, schools of nursing offering doctoral programs have assumed the arduous task of producing graduates who are experts in their specialty areas, and are both committed and able to advance nursing knowledge and practice through their research and leadership. Given these ambitious goals, as doctoral nursing education has matured it has become increasingly clear that the educational environment to which doctoral students are exposed is vitally important—perhaps even more than at any other educational level (Downs, 1988).

Doctoral students are not simply vessels into which faculty members pour their wisdom. In reality, they are eventually expected to become knowledge generators themselves. Therefore, these students require intense learning experiences in which they work hand-in-hand over a prolonged period with productive faculty researchers in order to become socialized as scholars. They must be imbued not only with these skills, but also with the norms and values of the scholar-researcher. Only in a positive scholarly environment in which the faculty display many of the characteristics of a community of scholars is successful socialization of developing scholars possible.

In this chapter, elements of a positive, growth-producing environment for a doctoral program are identified, with attention to individual, interpersonal, and institutional characteristics, as well as to linkages between the student and the environment. Factors that have been demonstrated empirically to contribute to and to impede positive environments are identified, and some strategies for optimizing environments suggested. Admittedly, the attempt to

75

identify characteristics of "optimal" or "positive" environments is a value-laden undertaking. Within the context of this chapter, the characteristics selected are either gleaned from empirical literature in graduate and nursing education or represent consensually validated standards or principles upon which judgments of quality are commonly based (Holzemer, 1982).

COMMUNITY OF SCHOLARS

The terminology that has commonly been used to epitomize a positive educational environment is "community of scholars." What is meant by this term? The dictionary definition of scholar refers to a learned individual who has profound knowledge of a selected field (Stein, 1969, p. 1277). Current usage within academia additionally incorporates the ideas that this expert remain abreast of current knowledge in the specialty and related fields; advance and effectively disseminate knowledge related to the specialty field through original research, theory building and testing, teaching, and publication; pursue professional activity and community service; is involved in the pursuit of excellence; is creative, curious, and actively engaged with novel ideas and activities; and is able to deal with abstractions (Copp, 1985b; Murphy, 1984; Pellino, Blackburn, & Boberg, 1984). Murphy (1984, p. 7) described the members of a community of scholars as vigorous; that is, they are ". . . energetically committed to and are exemplary in their provision of excellence in scholarship, research, teaching, and service to academia and to their profession."

The idea of a community of scholars not only signifies that there is a "critical mass" of individuals who meet the criteria for scholarship, but also suggests—consistent with the sociological conceptualization of community (Theodorson & Theodorson, 1969)—that these faculty share common traditions and interests, and constitute a social unit which is defined not by geographical space, but by a system of informal, interdependent relationships. Interpersonal relationships and special kinds of interaction patterns—characteristics that are additional to and different from those of the component members—are at the heart of being able to define an aggregate of scholarly individuals as a community of scholars.

In the kind of positive educational environment that is typified by the "community of scholars" label, faculty interact frequently and informally. Their interaction is not solely for the purpose of solving problems, nor is it limited to casual, superficial, or vacuous discussions. Rather, it is thoughtful, searching, and substantive; oriented toward acquiring and disseminating new knowledge. Conversations are often focused on scrutinizing and generating ideas and frequently cross disciplinary lines. In such an environment academic freedom with its attendant responsibilities, and a commitment to membership and participation in the growth and development of the university or college are apparent (Copp, 1985a).

A vital aspect of the ideal ". . . truly academic milieu, a company of scholars" (Copp, 1985b) is a sense of colleagiality and *esprit de corps*. That is:

Growth is encouraged, ideas are valued, scholarly activities are respected
. . . Students are seen as contributors; therefore, their opinions and questions
are sought. The success of a colleague, a superior or a novice is invested in by
all. Therefore, accomplishments are recognized and success is something in
which the group rejoices. Value is placed on the sense of self and the sense of
the common good of the school of nursing and the university (p. 188).

In such an environment faculty dare to be creative, to take risks in their thinking, to go out on intellectual limbs. They do not fear that their ideas will be
stolen or belittled, and are confident that peers will help them refine their
ideas. They do not hesitate to seek help or critical review of their work from
others, whose expertise they readily acknowledge and value. In fact, peer critique of ideas and of work completed and in progress is invited frequently. It is
given and accepted as constructive input, designed to improve the quality of
the work, and neither intended nor interpreted as a personal attack.

In a community of scholars consensus may be achieved about many aspects
of nursing, science, and philosophy, however, it is not necessarily expected,
nor is it required in order for progress to continue. Different perspectives and
opinions—even polar opposite positions—can exist simultaneously, be toler-
ated, and even encouraged as stimuli to intellectual ferment.

A community of scholars represents an "ideal type" of positive educational
environment. The combination of elements and characteristics which define
this ideal type may not all be present together to a high degree in any given
situation. They do represent desirable attributes, because they are consistent
with and conducive to high quality doctoral education.

FACULTY SCHOLARSHIP

Probably the most important component of any doctoral program is the
faculty, the basic elements or building blocks of a community of scholars. Because they serve as vital catalysts to student learning and primary agents for
socializing the scholar-researcher, doctoral faculty ideally are themselves scholars. Individuals who have not only earned the doctorate, but also are excited
by and continue to engage in significant postdoctoral knowledge-generating
activities, are those truly qualified to teach doctoral students. Although the
faculty role encompasses a wide variety of dimensions and activities (Andreoli
& Musser, 1986), scholarly productivity, as measured by involvement in research and numbers of funded (and unfunded) research projects and publications, is probably the most salient for doctoral level education. It is one of the
most commonly used indicators of doctoral faculty and program quality
(Holzemer, 1982; Holzemer and Chambers, 1986; AACN, 1987).

To date, few doctoral nursing programs have achieved the ideal that all
faculty teaching in the program are established scholars with ongoing research programs. The expectation that faculty engage in scholarship is relatively new in schools of nursing. As recently as 1984, Pellino and associates

cited findings that over half of full-time nurse faculty had published nothing or very little, and that 90 percent of the published articles were written by only 10 percent of faculty. However, in a more recent evaluation of doctoral nursing programs, in which productive faculty are likely to be concentrated, Holzemer and Chambers (1988) found that total career publications for faculty teaching in these programs averaged 18.4 (+17.6). Although the distribution of scholarly productivity remains concentrated in a relatively small handful of schools, it is rapidly evolving as an established norm in schools with graduate programs. Given its vital role in doctoral nursing education, it is important to identify the individual traits, background experiences, and work environments that seem to facilitate faculty productivity.

Individual Faculty Characteristics

Studies of productivity in a variety of academic disciplines suggest that several individual characteristics taken together seem to constitute the profile of a productive faculty member. Individuals whose academic, scholarly careers get off to an early start by virtue of having earned a doctorate and having begun publishing at an early age (generally before completing the doctoral degree), tend to be more productive throughout their careers than those who begin patterns of scholarship later in life. More productive faculty members also tend to have high motivation to publish, believe that publication is related to promotion, have a high level of interest in research, belong to selected professional organizations, and are in higher academic ranks (Bland & Schmitz, 1986; Holzemer & Chambers, 1988; Megel, Langston & Creswell, 1988; Ostmoe, 1986).

In general it has been found that women tend to publish at a lower rate than men, a problematic factor in trying to establish positive scholarly environments in schools of nursing. Many analysts, including those examining the low productivity of nurse faculty, have attributed women's lower productivity rate to role overload and conflict caused, in part, by competing demands placed on them in their roles as wives and mothers (Whitley, 1987; Whitley, Evans, Moody, Putnam, Sackett, & Vydareny, 1987). This explanation has been questioned by Cole and Zuckerman (1987) who found in a study of 120 non-nurse scientists that productivity fluctuated with changes in home and work responsibilities, but that the patterns were not directly related to marital status or motherhood.

Another explanation that has been advanced for female faculty members' lower productivity than their male counterparts' is that women have lacked mentors and sponsors to help socialize them to the expectations of the academic world (Clark and Corcoran, 1986; Whitley, 1987; Whitley, et al., 1987). Clark and Corcoran (1986) found that highly productive faculty had had the advantage of receiving a greater degree of sponsorship from their advisors than their less productive colleagues had had. In Bland and Schmitz's (1986) review of literature regarding faculty productivity, the productive researchers were likely to have received help and guidance from advisors or mentors before, during, and after their educational experiences. "Individuals who associate early with distinguished scientists or collaborate with them on research projects are more likely themselves to become productive researchers" (p. 24). One of the functions of a mentor is to help introduce the novice scholar to established investigators in the field. Continued interaction and networking with such individuals is a pattern which is characteristic of the productive researcher. A more detailed discussion of mentoring as a vital characteristic of a positive educational environment for a doctoral program is provided in a later section of the chapter.

Educational Preparation

The faculty member's educational preparation is seen to be a significant predictor of subsequent scholarly productivity (Blau, 1973). Not surprisingly, level of educational preparation relates directly to nurses' research and publication productivity (Hayter, 1984; Nieswiadomy, 1984; Ostmoe, 1986). The in-depth knowledge of a research area and mastery of methodological skills that are prerequisite to scholarly productivity are generally acquired at the doctoral level (Bland & Schmitz, 1986). Increasingly, postdoctoral research training is being advocated as a valuable underpinning for a research-oriented career in nursing, because of the extended period of experience and socialization it provides.

In their review of literature, Bland and Schmitz (1986) found that the nature of the researcher's educational preparation influenced future productivity in several ways. Productive researchers were highly socialized to the norms, expectations, and values of academia during their doctoral education, especially during the dissertation phase. Their educational experiences taught them what was expected of faculty members and helped inculcate the values of science and of the university professor role.

Many who have written about the success of nurses in faculty roles have argued that, when compared to their peers in other disciplines, nurse faculty may be at a disadvantage and may experience considerable role ambiguity and role conflict as faculty members (Batey, 1969; Fain, 1987, Megel, 1985; Williamson, 1972). These authors suggest that nurses' early socialization into the profession and the hospital setting inculcates norms that are antithetical to those that promote success in academia. Although Batey (1969) argued that graduate education does not provide sufficient opportunity for socialization in the skills, beliefs, and norms of scholarship; the situation in nursing has changed considerably in the last two decades. Many doctoral programs are indeed successful in resocializing nurses to faculty and scholar-researcher roles by providing opportunities to acquire values and behaviors associated with developing and disseminating new knowledge. Graduates of such programs should have little difficulty adjusting to faculty roles in settings where scholarship is valued and encouraged. In fact, they tend to become frustrated in environments where they cannot actualize their interest in research.

Time

The immediate work environment of the faculty member apparently has a considerable impact on scholarly productivity, one that is independent of individual ability and educational preparation. Time, an aspect of the work environment, is a concrete impediment or facilitator to scholarly productivity. Having (or making) sufficient time within the workload for research and publishing is a factor that seems to be a positive influence on faculty scholarly productivity (Megel, et al., 1988). This is true in both an absolute and a proportional sense. Clark, Corcoran, and Lewis (1986) studied faculty in 4 non-nursing fields and found that those who were rated most productive by their peers reported work weeks in excess of 60 hours. Holzemer and Chambers (1988) found that for faculty in doctoral nursing programs, the proportion of time spent in research and scholarship was the best predictor of scholarly productivity. Conversely, percentage of time spent in other components of the academic role, particularly clinical teaching, has been found to be inversely related to productivity rates (Ostmoe, 1986) and percentage of time spent in research (Holzemer & Chambers, 1988). Correspondingly, Coudret (1981) found that faculty with teaching loads greater than 20 hours per week reported difficulty in doing research.

It is difficult to determine from the existing literature whether low scholarly productivity is a necessary consequence of a heavy teaching load because of the time involved, or whether the relationship is spurious, due to a low level of interest in research. That is, a heavy time commitment to clinical teaching and relatively low productivity may both be attributable to the faculty member's level of interest in research and scholarship. Faculty members who place low priority on research may intentionally choose positions where teaching, rather than research, is prioritized and rewarded. Although the allocation of time to research is, in part, a function of administrative priority, faculty members—especially those teaching in graduate programs where clinical instruction loads are often lighter—may have considerable latitude to prioritize their time and plan their workloads accordingly. Those with high interest in research seem to be able to make time to do it.

Collegial Work Environment

The most pervasive finding from studies in many disciplines is that productivity seems to stimulate productivity. That is, faculty who work in an environment where scholarly productivity is high—or at least is perceived by them to be so—tend to be more productive in research and publication than those who work in settings with less productive peers (Braxton, 1983; Holzemer & Chambers, 1986, 1988). A given individual's productivity also seems to be highest in productive environments, implying that environmental characteristics may be every bit as important as those of the individual (Bland & Schmitz, 1986). Blau's (1973) study of academia revealed clearly that colleague climate, specifically "an academic environment of research-oriented colleagues" that promotes research involvement (p. 128), is the most important determinant of scholarly productivity.

> Whether an individual's research potentials become activated or suppressed depends in part on the colleague climate in his institution, specifically on the prevalency of research skills and orientations among colleagues, which stimulates his own research interests and exerts group pressures on him to engage in research (p. 128).

Holzemer and Chambers (1986, 1988) found nine interrelated environmental characteristics, taken as a group, to be associated with high faculty productivity. They included a supportive environment for learning, the perception of scholarly excellence, faculty concern for students, the variety and depth of the program offerings, the relevance and helpfulness of departmental procedures, availability of resources, student commitment and motivation, departmental direction and performance, and faculty satisfaction with departmental objectives and policies. Several of the most important factors that comprise and contribute to a positive doctoral program environment are examined below.

SUPPORTIVE RELATIONSHIPS

Supportive interpersonal professional relationships are a key ingredient for the kinds of positive educational environments that promote scholarly inquiry and research. A community of scholars is characterized by frequent and lively exchanges among faculty and students, informal interaction, open interchange, constructive critique of ideas, and tolerance and respect for pluralistic points of view. Advancing the view that a healthy doctoral program is one which combines balance, integration, and maximization of potential, Waltz (1985) characterized healthy doctoral program environments as reflecting several interpersonal characteristics that are analogous to those of a community of scholars. These include openness to new ideas and divergent points of view, mutual respect and concern between faculty and students and among faculty, a balance between academic freedom and concern for others' rights and needs, multiple opportunities for input and influence, encouragement for innovation and risk taking, awareness of and encouragement for the activities and accomplishments of others, and willingness to communicate one's thoughts and concerns directly. The extent to which these positive attributes exist varies from program to program and can change over time within the same institution.

In the health-related literature dealing with social support, the concept is used to designate helpful inputs that are received from and given to others in the individual's social network. Emotional inputs, including affirmation that one has worth and is cared for, and tangible help in the form of goods, services, and advice, are the major components of social support (Thoits, 1982). Just as social support has been found repeatedly to have beneficial effects on health, well-being, and performance, faculty scholars—even the most seasoned investigators—and doctoral students alike benefit from both emotional and tangible support from others in the educational environment. Within the context of doctoral education and faculty scholarship, emotional support would ideally enhance a sense of competence and self-confidence, convey that the faculty member (or student) is performing well and making a valued contribution to the institution or profession, and provide encouragement to pursue one's goals and ideas under adverse and frustrating conditions. Tangible support to the faculty scholar-researcher from peers most often consists of expert advice and suggestions, reviews that subject ideas and actions to scrutiny, and occasional concrete assistance with specific teaching, advisement, or research-related tasks. In his discussion of the impact of the collegial climate on faculty productivity, Blau (1973) emphasized the importance of supportive peer interaction and pointed out some of the mechanisms by which such interaction has a cumulatively beneficial effect within a faculty group.

> The discussion of such [research-active] colleagues about their research experiences—the problems encountered and the exciting discoveries made—with those who share research interests, and primarily with them, are incentives likely to activate any latent interest in research a person may have. To become a genuine member of a colleague group of this kind, one must be involved in research and thus be able to participate fully in the discussions about research. Colleagues with research skills facilitate one's own research by tending to give advice when needed, since being asked for advice is a welcome sign of respect for their superior skills, and they make working on research more gratifying by furnishing attentive listeners interested in hearing about promising leads and suggestive results. These processes of social exchange are a continued source of rewards for scholarly endeavors and create group pressures to engage in scholarly research by depriving those failing to do so of social rewards (p. 113).

One of the major deterrents to achieving a community of scholars is the fear of encountering an environment wherein interpersonal relationships are either apathetic or openly nonsupportive. In colleague groups where a majority of members or those in key formal or informal leadership positions are neither prepared for nor interested in research, normative pressures, including ridicule and lack of social approval, may stifle research interests (Blau, 1973). Unfortunately, even in environments where research is prevalent, lack of support for the scholarly efforts of individuals may be lacking. For example, dog-eat-dog competitiveness is not atypical of doctoral faculty in some institutions. Such patterns of interpersonal rivalry are accentuated by pressures to produce and scarcity of resources, including research funding and students (Brodie, 1986; Copp, 1985b). Whereas some degree of competition is a stimulus to productivity, continual one-upsmanship, backbiting, and territoriality are destructive and counterproductive to the doctoral program. They denigrate the accomplishments and worth of others, mitigate against the effective exchange of ideas and resources, and tend to pit subunits of a faculty group against one another unnecessarily. Similarly, "Queen Bee" behavior—involving excessive competition, elitism, and remoteness from others—precludes engaging in mutual critique and collaboration (May, Meleis, & Winstead-Fry, 1982).

Noting that subtle changes can diminish the health of a doctoral program's environment, Waltz (1985) discussed some indicators of ill health in doctoral program environments, particularly the interpersonal aspects:

1. Faculty–faculty and faculty–student contacts are limited to formal settings.

2. There is a notable absence of students and faculty, except when classes necessitate their being present.

3. Students and faculty are unaware of the research endeavors of others in the setting.

4. A preponderance of communication is written rather than face-to-face.

5. Some faculty are unwilling to serve with others on students' committees.

6. Students and faculty hesitate to express their concerns directly to those involved.

7. Faculty are unable to resolve issues satisfactorily without repeatedly resurrecting them.

8. Contacts with scholars outside the department and school are very limited.

In such an environment relationships are highly utilitarian and potentially exploitive, hardly consistent with the supportive colleague climate that typifies a community of scholars.

Collaboration

One of the most effective means for fostering not only scholarly productivity, but also a supportive personal environment is to institute collaborative research projects and other scholarly activities. Collaboration has the advantages of blending the efforts of faculty with complementary expertise, providing an excellent arena for junior faculty to learn from those more experienced in scholarly inquiry, and providing a reasonable division of labor for carrying out time-consuming research projects. Strategies that have been used intramurally to promote collaborative research and scholarship include establishing research interest groups to address areas of mutual interest, establishing journal clubs to discuss state-of-the-art advances in the field, actively recruiting faculty with common interests to engage in planning a cluster of related research projects, and stipulating that collaboration is a necessary condition for receiving institutional research funds. One of the exciting advantages of collaborative research is that, following an initial joint undertaking, the collaborators often go on to conduct "offspring" projects on their own or with other investigators. The results produce a "snowball effect" on the level of interest in and enthusiasm for scholarship and on the number of faculty involved in research and cumulative knowledge building in the substantive area of the research (Gioiella, 1985; Lenz, 1987; Pender, Sechrist, Frank-Stromborg & Walker, 1987; Pollock, 1986).

Mentoring

Although a range of supportive relationships have been identified in academic settings (e.g., peer pal, sponsor, advisor, educator, "boss"), the one currently receiving the most attention is the mentor–protégé relationship. Defined in a variety of ways, mentorship is generally considered to be an intense and relatively long-term relationship between a novice in a discipline (or organization) and a more influential authority or expert, who is also higher on the career and organizational ladder (Allen, 1986; May, et al., 1982). Mentoring is said to differ from other supportive relationships, in that it involves more than guidance, counsel, and imparting knowledge. A commitment is made by the mentor to the person's total intellectual and professional growth. The student's independence as a scholar and relationships with other noted scholars are actively promoted (Fitzpatrick & Abraham, 1987; May, et al., 1982).

The mentor–protégé relationship is currently being advocated as an effective means to socialize new faculty and graduate students to the scholar-researcher and faculty roles (Allen, 1986; Bogat & Redner, 1985; Fitzpatrick & Abraham, 1987; Megel, 1985). Benefits accrue primarily to the student, who receives guidance, opportunities to share ideas with an expert in the field, assistance with developing leadership and research skills, indoctrination to the institute's politics and expectations, help with "learning the ropes" of the job and the institution, and opportunities to make valuable professional connections. The mentor, in addition to gaining a sense of personal fulfillment, can benefit from a jointly productive relationship, particularly when scholarly collaboration is involved.

Both Pollock (1986) and Allen (1986) have noted that the institution and the profession can also benefit when mentorship is prevalent in the educational environment. Pollock (1986) found that in top-ranked schools of nursing, junior faculty were attracted by the potential opportunity to work closely with experienced nurse researchers. Allen (1986) argued that mentorship benefits the institution and profession by developing talent, providing continuity, and encouraging the self-confidence and knowledge needed for leadership.

The mentor–protégé relationship begins with a clearly unequal distribution of power. Initially the student is an apprentice who is learning and being assisted. At later stages the relationship ideally evolves into one of collegiality, wherein the student is an independent contributor (Megel, 1985). Potential dangers of the mentor–protégé relationship are that the student may become and remain subservient or overly dependent on, overly protected, or exploited by the mentor. The result is that creativity—and ultimately opportunity and contribution—are stifled. The relationship may be so intense that the student becomes isolated from peers and other senior members of the faculty whose views happen to differ from those of the mentor. This results in restricted exposure to alternative perspectives. To avoid such problems, May, Meleis, and Winstead-Fry (1982) recommended that a student or junior faculty member seek several mentors over the course of doctoral study and the early postdoctoral career. Mentorship cannot be mandated or assigned. Some senior faculty enjoy and are exceptionally skilled at mentoring novice scholars, whereas other lack the patience, time, or interest to do so. According to May, et al. (1982), the ideal mentorship for scholarliness is based on the mentor's being actively involved in scholarly inquiry and research, conceptually sound, willing to discuss ideas and options with the student, self-confident, and capable and willing to provide guidance. The prospective protégé must be open to mentorship, "capable of adult intimacy" (p. 27), eager to be socialized into scholarly roles, and willing to listen to advice. Those junior faculty who seek mentorship are advised to participate in activities that bring them into contact with potential mentors; for example, joining committees or research teams headed by senior faculty and engaging in discussions of common substantive interests or professional issues with senior faculty (Megel, et al., 1988).

ADMINISTRATIVE SUPPORT

The active support of top- and middle-level administrators is clearly vital in encouraging faculty productivity and a positive educational climate (Pollock, 1986). Administrative support for research can take many forms. In Blau's (1973) view, possibly the most important thing an administrator can do is to recruit and hire qualified, research-prepared, and productive faculty. Although they command high salaries, productive scholars have the effect of creating a collegial climate that further catalyzes scholarly productivity. Additionally, they are likely to have a cosmopolitan orientation, multiple ties to scholars in other institutions, and high visibility in the profession and the larger scientific community. Such characteristics not only help place them—and ideally the colleagues with whom they work closely—in the professional mainstream, but also expose them to state-of-the-art knowledge in their fields of interest. The presence of known and visible scholars on a faculty also acts as a magnet to attract additional high quality faculty at both junior and senior levels (Murphy, 1984).

Administrators can influence the scholarly productivity of faculty through their input regarding merit, promotion and tenure criteria, policies, and decisions. Certainly they can and should be explicit about their expectations that faculty engage in research and publication, and can back up their expectations with sanctions. For example, merit salary increases can be predicated on research involvement or securing external research funding. In tenure and promotion criteria, universities with graduate programs tend to weight research more heavily than do colleges that are oriented primarily to undergraduate education. Blau (1973) argued, on the basis of his classic study of higher education, that such policies do not serve as major incentives to faculty research, but help screen faculty and encourage those who are research-oriented to select a particular institution. Although the screening function operates in nursing as well, it is probable that recent changes in criteria for promotion and tenure have a direct effect on increasing the overall productivity rate of nursing faculty, particularly those in schools with doctoral programs.

All school of nursing administrators surveyed by Kruger and Washburn (1987) considered research to be an important basis for promotion and tenure decisions, and nearly all (98%) rated teaching to be important as well. Their opinions were consistent with Blau's (1973) position that both teaching and research responsibilities are crucial and should be emphasized in graduate education, even though it results in heavy role demands on faculty. To the extent that they back up their beliefs in the importance of research for merit, promotion, and tenure with concrete rewards and workload assignments, administrators can be instrumental in fostering positive, productive educational environments for their doctoral programs.

Top- and middle-level administrators' attitudes and actions can help set the tone for the doctoral program's faculty and students. For example, Gioiella (1985) described the things she had done as a new dean to help promote research and scholarship in a baccalaureate program. Lack of encouragement had been cited as a barrier to productivity, so she launched a "campaign of concentrated positive reinforcement for scholarly productivity" (p. 258) by frequently and avidly articulating a message of pride in the faculty and its accomplishments and potential. She was also instrumental in establishing a research interest group whose activities ultimately resulted in a grant submission.

In some cases deans and department chairpersons are also exerting informal influence through role-modeling scholarly behaviors. A number of individuals currently holding administrative positions in schools of nursing and high positions in universities established themselves as eminent scholars well before they became administrators. Many continue extensive, externally funded research programs while carrying out administrative responsibilities—not an easy task, but one that clearly demonstrates their commitment to scholarship.

While their encouragement and facilitation certainly plays a role in stimulating faculty scholarship, the relative importance of administrative support is not clear. Blau's (1973) findings suggest that it is much less important than the collegial climate, which is, in turn, influenced greatly by the structural characteristics of the university. Wakefield-Fisher (1987) found that deans' leadership styles, measured in terms of their task and relationship orientation, had no impact on the scholarly productivity of the faculty in doctoral nursing programs. On the other hand, it is easy to speculate that a highly controlling or nonsupportive administrator—one who does not value research and may actively discourage faculty from pursuing it—could have a very negative influence on a doctoral program's environment by providing deterrents that would cause research-committed faculty to leave or reduce their scholarly output.

Both positive and negative administrative behavior were deemed to be major supportive and hindering factors, respectively, by faculty in several departments of a major midwestern university (Clark, Corcoran, & Lewis, 1986).

SUPPORT FACILITIES AND SERVICES FOR RESEARCH

One of the ways in which administrators can actively encourage a positive, research-oriented environment for a doctoral program is to take steps to assure that faculty with an interest in research have adequate facilities and services available to them. Needed facilities include computer hardware and software, research libraries, and access to laboratory space and equipment for both physiological and psychosocial research. Such laboratory facilities, if not available within the school of nursing, can often be borrowed or rented from basic science departments. Faculty input regarding equipment and facilities requirements for such laboratories is crucial. Space to house graduate student research assistants or the staff for a funded project is a frequently overlooked resource that often must be negotiated repeatedly as research activities increase in schools that were once almost totally consumed by the teaching function of the faculty.

Services that are necessary to support the research activities of faculty often require considerable financial commitments. They include secretarial service; expert consultation regarding research design, statistics, grant writing and computer programming; bibliographic searches; hands-on assistance with data collection and analysis; help in locating potential funding sources; equipment maintenance and repair; editing; and preparation of graphics for publications and presentations. Although not services per se, institutional funds to support small scale pilot or preliminary studies and to help subsidize faculty travel to professional meetings to make presentations and remain up to date in the field of their research, can have a considerable impact on scholarly productivity. Administrators' priorities determine, to a great extent, the funding that is allocated to such research support.

Research Centers

One of the prevalent patterns in schools of nursing has been to designate a research center or similar structure to facilitate faculty and student research. Research centers or offices in top-rated schools (Pollock, 1986) and schools of nursing in general (McArt, 1987) typically provide consultation, assistance with grant preparation, computer services, reference materials, peer review of manuscripts and proposals, and information dissemination about meetings and funding opportunities. With both rising concerns about the ethical dimensions of nursing research and problems of research fraud and academic misconduct occurring in some disciplines, research centers may increasingly be asked to provide consultation on the ethics of research and scholarship. Perhaps one of their most valuable functions is to heighten the visibility of research as a legitimate and high priority activity within the school. To the extent that research center staff (primarily the director who is often an active and productive nurse researcher) exhibit enthusiasm about research and role model scholarly productivity, their existence can act as a vital catalyst to a positive climate for scholarship.

The pattern of establishing a separate structural unit to facilitate research and to provide needed support is relatively uncommon in academic departments other than professional schools, such as nursing and social work. Although the demand for such centers has grown with increases in the number of nurses with doctorates, the question of whether the need for them will continue as nurse faculty become more sophisticated and experienced researchers has been raised (McArt, 1987). Although some leading schools with doctoral programs have phased out their research centers, they remain a valuable resource for faculty groups that have not evolved to the point where research and scholarly productivity are institutionalized.

Endowed Chairs

Currently there are few endowed professorships or research chairs within nursing. However, it has been argued that establishing such a chair can be a tremendous incentive for scholarship and a considerable research support resource for a school of nursing. McNeely, Moody, and Anderson (1987) maintained that establishing an endowed chair is a university's ultimate form of legitimation for a discipline. It allows a school or department to increase the visibility of its disciplinary research to the public, as well as to other units of the university. It also encourages advancement of research efforts in a focused area, and helps socialize upcoming scholars. Because endowed chairs are usually filled by noted scholars, they can help attract well-qualified students and junior faculty to the school. They can also generate increased research funding as the incumbent secures grants or inspires others to seek extramural funding for their research programs. Because of the prestige associated with it, the endowed chair is an excellent and highly visible way for an institution to reward demonstrated scholarly productivity.

LINKING THE STUDENT AND THE ENVIRONMENT

If the educational environment is to have an impact on the doctoral student, they must be linked together. As with any contextual analysis, it is important to consider the strength of the tie between the environment and the individual or group whose behavior is being explained. For example, the impact of a religious sect's doctrine is greatest for those members who are tied most strongly to it through frequent church attendance and participation in multiple religious activities. By extension, then, one may argue that the impact of a positive educational environment on students is variable, depending on the strength of the ties linking the student to it.

An important indicator of the strength of the link between the doctoral program environment and the student is whether enrollment is full time;

enrollment status is a proxy indicator for the amount of time the student is actually exposed to environmental influences. It seems evident that the more time and attention students devote to their doctoral studies in a given year, and the fewer distractions and diversions they experience, the stronger their ties to the program. Students who "drop in" for a course each semester over a period of seven or eight years and spend little time interacting with peers and faculty would be minimally influenced by the program's environment, regardless of how positive it may be. Conversely, students who are able to immerse themselves in the program's subculture forge multifaceted links to the environment and are likely to be impacted by it.

In their discussion of ways to socialize future scientists in PhD programs, Fitzpatrick and Abraham (1987) recommended a model of doctoral education that calls for faculty integration of students in their research throughout the students' doctoral study. The techniques they suggest for such integration provide students with increasing responsibility as they progress through the program. Students become socialized by spending time in discussions with faculty and fellow students, attending and participating in seminars, serving as research assistants on faculty research projects, and even directing small-scale studies that are closely aligned with the faculty member's research program. In this integrative model students are involved not only in the more technical "doing" aspects of research, but also in the conceptual, issue-oriented "thinking" aspects. The model is time- and energy-consuming for student and faculty member alike, but ultimately benefits both, as well as the program as a whole.

Student–Faculty and Peer Relations

The primary mechanism by which student–environment links are formed and strengthened is the student–faculty relationship. Doctoral students, when surveyed about the most important elements in their graduate environments, noted faculty–student relationships (which had both negative and positive elements) as most important. Second in importance was the extent to which the department was a true community (Harnett, 1976). Bargar and Mayo-Chamberlain (1983), emphasizing the advisor–advisee relationship, advocated a pattern whereby the advisor would remain constructively involved with the student throughout the entire program and beyond. They urged faculty advisors to express interest in the student's work and welfare; encourage open discussion of issues with the student; help students to develop incisiveness, creativity, independent problem solving, and the ability to be self-critical. Positive relationships with the faculty help students view themselves as proactive shapers of their educational environment. Because the relationship is to be reciprocal, the students share equal responsibility for maintaining open, trusting communication with their advisors.

Bargar and Mayo-Chamberlain's (1983) recommendations about the activities an advisor should perform in a positive, developmentally-oriented relationship parallel many included by Fitzpatrick and Abraham (1987) in their description of mentorship. However, being an advisor to a doctoral student does not require that the faculty member serve as a mentor in the full sense of the term. Faculty other than the advisor can mentor a student; and students should feel free to develop positive relationships with a number of faculty members. Not all advisor–advisee relationships are ideal. Mismatches should be rectified quickly and without prejudice, so that each student's links to the program's environment can be maximized.

In addition to faculty, students' peers can help provide linkages to the doctoral program environment. Students in a dynamic program learn as much from one another as from the faculty. They become accustomed to receiving review and critique of their ideas from their fellow students. More advanced students serve as role models and informants to those at earlier stages of doctoral study. Such relationships are facilitated by providing a designated space for doctoral students to meet informally and by faculty-initiated activities, such as seminars and social gatherings.

TOWARD DOCTORAL FACULTY AS A COMMUNITY OF SCHOLARS

The challenge to today's doctoral nursing programs is to produce tomorrow's knowledge builders and leaders. A program's ability to produce nurse scholars and scientists depends considerably on the extent to which its environment is conducive to, and in fact demands, high quality scholarship. On the basis of the foregoing analysis, it is clear that the beliefs and actions of faculty and administrators create the positive environments that are crucial to high quality doctoral education.

Faculty must be scholars themselves if they expect to engender enthusiasm for scholarship in their students. They must actively integrate students in their research, and commit the time and energy to serve as mentors to help socialize junior faculty members and students to the scholar-researcher role. Notably, if members of a faculty are to become a community of scholars, they must move beyond a focus on themselves and their own productivity to broader concern with the scholarship of the group as a whole. Commitment to the faculty as a community places emphasis on collegiality, mutual support, and stimulation. Commitment to socializing students means that research interests and activities must be balanced by exquisite teaching and willingness to work closely in collaboration with students and colleagues.

Administrative commitment to scholarship and research is a crucial underpinning for a doctoral program. It helps determine the characteristics of faculty recruited, the priority placed on scholarly productivity in the formal reward structure and in faculty workload, the visibility of the institution's commitment to scholarship, and the resources allocated to stimulate and support faculty research efforts. Just as administrators help set the tone for the degree of research emphasis in a program's environment, they can also be instrumental in fostering intellectual ferment, collaboration, collegiality, and mutual respect, rather than excessive internal competition within the faculty.

To approximate a community of scholars is a considerable achievement for a doctoral program faculty, one that is undoubtedly well worth the great effort involved. After all, doctoral education is an expensive undertaking for students, faculty, and institutions. The probability that the expense will represent energy, time, and money well spent depends, in large part, on the quality and health of the educational environment.

REFERENCES

Allen, D. S. (1986). Promoting professional career development: A case for mentors. *Educational Directions, 11* (3), 25-31.

American Association of Colleges of Nursing. (1987). Indicators of quality in doctoral programs in nursing. *Journal of Professional Nursing, 3,* 72-74.

Andreoli, K. G., & Musser, L. A. (1986). Faculty productivity. In H. H. Werley, J. J. Fitzpatrick, & R. L. Taunton (Eds.), *Annual Review of Nursing Research* (Vol. 4) (pp. 177-193). New York: Springer Publishing.

Bargar, R. R., & Mayo-Chamberlain, J. (1983). Advisor and advisee issues in doctoral education. *Journal of Higher Education, 54,* 407-432.

Batey, M. V. (1969). The two normative worlds of the university nursing faculty. *Nursing Forum, 8,* 4-16.

Bland, C. J., & Schmitz, C. C. (1986). Characteristics of the successful researcher and implications for faculty development. *Journal of Medical Education, 61,* 22-31.

Blau, P. (1973). *The organization of academic work.* New York: Wiley.

Bogat, G. A., & Redner, R. L. (1985). How mentoring affects the professional development of women in psychology. *Professional Psychology: Research and Practice, 16,* 851-859.

Braxton, J. M. (1983). Department colleagues and individual faculty productivity. *Review of Higher Education, 6,* 125-128.

Brodie, B. (1986). Impact of doctoral programs on nursing education. *Journal of Professional Nursing, 2,* 350-357.

Clark, S. M., & Corcoran, M. (1986). Perspectives on the professional socialization of women faculty: A case of cumulative disadvantage. *Journal of Higher Education, 57,* 20-43.

Clark, S. M., Corcoran, M., & Lewis, D. R. (1986). The case for an institutional perspective on faculty development. *Journal of Higher Education, 57*(2), 176-195.

Cole, J. R., & Zuckerman, H. (1987). Marriage, motherhood and research performance in science. *Scientific American, 256,* 119-125.

Copp, L. A. (1985a). Becoming a faculty member. *Journal of Professional Nursing, 1,* 259, 317.

Copp, L. A. (1985b). The colleague relationship. *Journal of Professional Nursing, 1,* 144.

Coudret, N. A. (1981). Determining faculty workload. *Nurse Educator, 6*(2), 38-41.

Downs, F. S. (1988). Doctoral education: Our claim to the future. *Nursing Outlook, 36,* 18-20.

Fain, J. A. (1987). Perceived role conflict, role ambiguity, and job satisfaction among nurse educators. *Journal of Nursing Education, 26,* 223-238.

Fitzpatrick, J. J., & Abraham, I. L. (1987). Toward the socialization of scholars and scientists. *Nurse Educator, 12*(3), 23-25.

Gioiella, E. C. (1985). Promoting research among baccalaureate program faculty members: A success story. *Journal of Professional Nursing, 1,* 258, 317.

Harnett, R. T. (1976). Environments for advanced learning. In J. Katz & R. T. Harnett (Eds.), *Scholars in the Making* (pp. 49-84). Cambridge: Ballinter.

Hayter, J. (1984). Institutional sources of articles published in 13 nursing journals. *Nursing Research, 33,* 357-362.

Holzemer, W. L. (1982). Quality in graduate nursing education. *Nursing & Health Care, 3,* 536-542.

Holzemer, W. L., & Chambers, D. B. (1986). Healthy nursing doctoral programs: Relationship between perceptions of the academic environment and productivity of faculty and alumni. *Research in Nursing and Health, 9,* 299-307.

Holzemer, W. L., & Chambers, D. B. (1988). A contextual analysis of faculty productivity. *Journal of Nursing Education, 27,* 10-18.

Kruger, S., & Washburn, J. (1987). Tenure and promotion: An update on university nursing faculty. *Journal of Nursing Education, 26,* 182-188.

Lawrence, J. H., & Blackburn, R. T. (1985). Faculty careers: Maturation, demographic and historical effects. *Research in Higher Education, 22,* 135-155.

Lenz, E. R. (1987). Strategies for developing and implementing a focused research effort. *Nursing Outlook, 35,* 60-64.

May, K. M., Meleis, A. I., & Winstead-Fry, P. (1982). Mentorship for scholarliness: Opportunities and dilemmas. *Nursing Outlook, 30,* 22-26.

McArt, E. W. (1987). Research facilitation in academic and practice settings. *Journal of Professional Nursing, 3,* 84-91.

McNeely, J. B., Moody, L. E., & Anderson, G. C. (1987). Endowed research chairs: Perceptions from other disciplines and implications for the nursing scientific community. *Journal of Professional Nursing, 3,* 114-117.

Megel, M. E. (1985). New faculty in nursing: Socialization and the role of the mentor. *Journal of Nursing Education, 24,* 303-306.

Megel, M. E., Langston, N. F., & Creswell, J. W. (1988). Scholarly productivity: A survey of nursing faculty researchers. *Journal of Professional Nursing, 4,* 45–54.

Murphy, J. F. (1984). Essential resources for developing a doctoral program in nursing. *Nurse Educator, 9*(4), 6–10.

Nieswiadomy, R. M. (1984). Nurse educators' involvement in research. *Journal of Nursing Education, 23,* 52–56.

Ostmoe, P. M. (1986). Correlates of university nurse faculty publication productivity. *Journal of Nursing Education, 25,* 207–212.

Pellino, G. R., Blackburn, R. T., & Boberg, A. L. (1984). The dimensions of academic scholarship: Faculty and administrator views. *Research in Higher Education, 20,* 103–115.

Pender, N. J., Sechrist, K. R., Frank-Stromborg, M., & Walker, S. N. (1987). Collaboration in developing a research program grant. *Image, 19,* 75–77.

Pollock, S. E. (1986). Top-ranked schools of nursing: Network of scholars. *Image, 18,* 58–60.

Stein, J. (Ed.). (1969). *The Random House Dictionary of the English Language.* New York: Random House.

Solomons, H. C., Jordison, N. S., & Powell, S. R. (1980). How faculty members spend their time. *Nursing Outlook, 28,* 160–165.

Theodorson, G. A., & Theodorson, A. G. (1969). *Modern dictionary of sociology.* New York: Thomas Y. Crowell.

Thoits, P. A. (1982). Conceptual, methodological, and theoretical problems in studying social support as a buffer against life stress. *Journal of Health and Social Behavior, 23,* 145–159.

Wakefield-Fisher, M. (1987). The relationship between professionalization of nursing faculty, leadership styles of deans and faculty scholarly productivity. *Journal of Professional Nursing, 3,* 155–164.

Waltz, C. F. (1985). What is a healthy doctoral program? A faculty perspective. In K. Brown (Ed.), *Proceedings of the Ninth Forum on Doctoral Education in Nursing* (pp. 170–180). Birmingham: University of Alabama.

Whitley, N. O. (1987). Women in academic radiology. *American Journal of Radiology, 149,* 438–439.

Whitley, N. O., Evans, R. G., Moody, M. A., Putnam, C. E., Sackett, J. F., & Vydareny, K. H. (1987). Advancement of women in academic radiology. *Investigative Radiology, 22,* 431–436.

Williamson, J. A. (1972). The conflict-producing role of the professionally socialized nurse-faculty member. *Nursing Forum, 9,* 357–366.

6

Readiness Assessment: Asking and Answering the Critical Questions

Mary E. Conway, PhD, FAAN

The recent proliferation of doctoral programs in a variety of disciplines is a reflection of both competition and a move toward diversity—particularly in large multi-purpose universities. Competition, whether overt or covert, is fundamentally a race for ever scarcer resources, especially for extramural funds and, to a lesser extent, for graduate students. Newer roles in an increasingly diversified economy are expected to provide jobs for those with a doctoral degree even if the doctorate is not a requisite for the job in question (Mayhew & Ford, 1974). In this overall picture the case for nursing is somewhat different; it has taken nursing as a professional discipline considerably longer to establish the prevalence of the doctorate than other fields. Thus, while an overabundance of PhDs is predicted for the 1990s, a shortage of nurse doctorates has been forecast (U.S. Institute of Medicine, 1983). While some decry what appears to be a race to establish doctoral programs in nursing—often without the requisite base in faculty and other resources—the "race" can quite properly be viewed as a rational response to a data-based forecast of future demand.

The purpose of this chapter is to explore what constitutes readiness to initiate a doctoral program in nursing. In undertaking this exploration comments will be directed specifically to PhD programs. While many of the factors that will be identified as requisite to supporting a quality doctoral program would apply equally to the professional doctorate (DNS or other), not all would. One example of a requisite that applies more specifically to the PhD program is a strong research base provided by incumbent faculty; one that would apply to both is the existence of a large library collection and mainframe and satellite computer capability.

95

A PERSPECTIVE

Before attempting to identify specific factors which indicate that a particular university is ready to start a new doctoral program in any discipline, it may be useful to shape a perspective which will dictate the salient factors to be considered.

The movement toward establishment of doctoral programs in nursing (32 additional programs initiated between 1978 and 1987) is counter to the trend toward retrenchment in many institutions of higher education (National League for Nursing, 1988). In fact, seeking approval for a doctoral program may be coincident with internal reassessment and/or retrenchment in the same university. In discussing internal reassessment, Mingle and Norris (1981) outline 7 criteria for the evaluation of existing academic programs which should be considered prior to a decision to continue or discontinue any one of them. Several of their criteria are extremely relevant to the consideration of initiating a new doctoral program in nursing. While Mingle and Norris discuss internal reassessment involving an entire university, the practical consequences of initiating a single new program—in the absence of total reassessment—are identical in one respect: new programs come at the expense of existing programs. The following 5 criteria are particularly relevant when considering the possibility of starting a new program: essentiality of the new program to the university, potential quality of the program, need for the program, demand (in the employment market), and cost implications. In this chapter essentiality of program and cost are discussed at some length under the heading of political and fiscal factors. Both need and demand are clearly well established (U.S. Department of Health and Human Services, 1988).

The Council of Graduate Schools of the United States has published a small monograph which captures the essence of doctoral study (Council of Graduate Schools, 1977). The central purpose of study leading to the doctor of philosophy degree is the extension of knowledge. Students engaged in doctoral study are expected to "evaluate critically the literature in the field and to apply appropriate principles and procedures to the recognition, evaluation, interpretation, and understanding of issues and problems at the frontiers of knowledge" (p. 1). One feature of a superior program is the presence of other strong doctoral programs on the same campus which can allow students an opportunity for a minor field in order to "provide breadth as well as depth of training" (p. 2). Additional characteristics of the optimal environment for doctoral study include a well-qualified faculty who are experts in their profession or field of science; are committed to graduate education and to the graduate student; and, in the aggregate, have a commitment to their respective departments. Beyond the departmental level, administrative officials and an administrative structure which is enthusiastic about graduate study are a *sine qua non* for quality programs.

The foregoing description is a "recipe" for success. In the aggregate the factors emphasized form a set of criteria against which an institution and its decisionmakers can assess their readiness to mount a doctoral program. The process of assessment requires a degree of honesty that may be hard to come by in the eagerness to start a new program. A commonly expressed justification on the part of university officials about to begin a new venture is that the venture will help further the mission of the university—or school, or department. While such a justification in itself cannot be faulted, an obscuring cloud of self-interest will not be beneficial. A strong argument could be made that any number of new or innovative programs would further the mission of the university, but each such initiative should be measured against the welfare of the entire institution and its constituent parts. For example, what programs must be foregone if the one under consideration is mounted? Will the almost certain necessity for reallocation of resources work to the detriment of some other school or department? If a timetable for development has been outlined, would a slowing of the timetable result in any serious harm; or, might it allow for more equitable development and strengthening of other parts of the system? Each institution and its representatives is likely to differ in the answers to these questions. Disciplinary loyalty, departmental loyalty, "star" performers— each represent forces which must be considered. The internal view is likely to be biased and even distorted; thus, an evaluation of the situation by external experts can be a great help in approaching the eventual internal decision. Any responsible assessment of readiness to mount a doctoral program must also take into account decreasing enrollments and lowered public support; the latter reflected in "hold steady" allocations for public institutions of higher education (Baldridge, Curtis, Ecker, & Riley, 1978; p. 205).

Given this general perspective on some basic essentials underpinning strong graduate programs, what core factors need to be considered? At least five general categories within which salient factors can be grouped are:

1. Environment—including political and fiscal factors

2. The academic milieu

3. Research capability

4. Faculty

5. Physical facilities

SALIENT FACTORS IN ASSESSING READINESS

The Environment

Political and fiscal factors. Consideration of the environment and its anticipated contribution to or restraint of a new program involves taking both a systems and a local perspective. (A system's perspective may be less critical to a private university than to a public one.) Within the environmental perspective both the academic climate and the fiscal climate must be examined.

In dealing with a school or college of nursing located in a public university, it is vital to know how much priority is given to nursing as an academic discipline in the state's overall plan. In a state where a large number of nursing programs exist, nursing may not be strongly supported with respect to the allocation of resources. Allocations may be thinly spread across all schools. On the other hand, if the state supports one or more large health care facilities, nursing may command a high priority. If this is true, it is reasonable to expect that a doctoral program, if well planned and justified, is likely to gain both approval and sufficient funding to ensure a sound start-up.

One area that needs to be dealt with cautiously is that of presumed priorities. Published statements of support for nursing—or any other discipline—by the Regents or Chancellor of a system may be quite distinct from the political realities of funding. In many states the Regents are charged with outlining standards, priorities, and long-range growth of the higher education system while the legislature holds the purse strings. If the legislature historically underfunds Regents' proposals, or, if there are serious political conflicts, chances for securing the additional funds needed to initiate a new program are minimal.

However thoughtful the appraisal of the environment in higher education in a given region or state, it is impossible to accurately predict what public policy will be in the near or distant future in the area of funding higher education. One respected source calls this the "zone of uncertainty" (Carnegie Foundation for the Advancement of Teaching, 1975). The Carnegie authors further state, "The effects on higher education of possible changes in public policy toward student aid, institutional aid, graduate education and research are probably more important than all the other uncertainties combined" (p. 48).

Still another factor that must be considered is the overall master plan of the system. Which disciplines are slated for growth? Which for holding steady or phase out?

Priorities as reflected in master plans or other documents, as well as political considerations are factors of great importance in assessing the possibilities for program approval and both short-and long-range fiscal support for a new program. A number of private universities may be handicapped by a shrinking base of undergraduate students enrolled in nursing—a trend of the recent past. A large undergraduate base offers fiscal support to a doctoral program in that, generally, the larger the undergraduate enrollment, the larger the faculty size. Thus, an initial expansion which commits more faculty hours and effort to doctoral students is unlikely to have a deleterious effect on undergraduate teaching. When the initial impact on faculty effort and teaching assignments is low, there is opportunity for the dean or administrator to plan with reasonable lead time for securing additional funds and/or reallocating funds which are reasonably certain to be available.

Another consideration in a multicampus system is the extent to which intercampus cooperation/collaboration is encouraged. A trend in recent years is the move toward more interschool cooperation with the specific aims of nonduplication of expensive programs and a broader sharing of faculty resources. For example, while three or four colleges in a large university system may offer graduate courses in physics, only the flagship school may have an internationally renowned expert in nuclear physics on its faculty. Thus, a cooperative program might be in place which allows students to register at several campuses during the course of graduate study in order to take advantage of the expertise found in the various schools or colleges.

In a public system of higher education where a precedent for cooperative degree programs exists, early exploration of the possibilities for the establishment of such a program leading to the PhD in nursing would be well advised.

What is important to bear in mind is that whatever the fiscal and/or political climate may be, strategies specific to *that* environment can and should be outlined. Raising public opinion to the desirability and need of a doctoral program in nursing is one strategy that can be used to good advantage in almost every situation. The obvious value of nursing to society is a plus in the realm of public opinion. A school (and faculty) that can draw a clear connection between excellence in practice and the existence of a corps of researchers and master teachers whose combined efforts are directed toward enhancing excellence in practice can make a strong case in winning support for a doctoral program. Getting the message *to* the public can be a challenge in itself. Being politically sensitive to what are acceptable means of getting the message into the media is all important in determining the eventual success or failure.

The Academic Milieu

An important question that should be asked when contemplating a doctoral program in nursing is what the strength is of the graduate school. Is it a visible force in setting and monitoring standards for curriculum, dissertation committees, research activities, and progression? In rare instances a particular graduate school may not have a national reputation for excellence while the school of nursing may enjoy prominence. However, the better the reputation of the graduate school, the more drawing power will exist for attracting top quality students to the doctoral program in nursing.

As noted earlier the presence of strong graduate programs in other disciplines is an essential adjunct for the doctoral program in nursing. While the core curriculum and research are focused in nursing, doctoral students need access to scholars and researchers in allied fields such as physiology, philosophy, ethics, biology, sociology, and psychology. In fact, many graduate schools require the candidate for the PhD to have a faculty member outside his own discipline on the dissertation committee. Strong programs of study in other disciplines allow the doctoral nurse student to select cognate courses which support the selected area of specialization or research. In some universities the nurse is encouraged to select a minor area of concentration such as developmental psychology or ethics, for example. Interdisciplinary symposia conducted periodically add intellectual enrichment to the total program of study for all students.

A further academic quality measure is related to the success of past and present doctoral candidates in the university. What is the completion record of all doctoral candidates? How many pass or fail the qualifying examinations? Do a large number of students who have been admitted to candidacy leave the university ABD? Assuming that students are carefully selected for admission initially, the completion rate across disciplines is a meaningful indicator of program quality.

Research Capability

Research and/or research potential of the university as a whole is an absolute imperative for any doctoral program. Schools differ in their research prominence and the amount of resources devoted to research. Because every university does not have an equal capacity or track record in research, it is very difficult to judge the status of research in a given institution. One solid indicator of research emphasis—as well as potential for further development—is the recent historical record. The record will contain the total amount of intramural dollars allocated to research over past years, the amount of extramural dollars generated by faculty research, the total number of faculty actively engaged in research, the number of faculty who serve (or have served) on NIH study sections, and the amount of space allocated to research projects. An annual listing of faculty publications will provide further evidence of research productivity.

The school of nursing planning to have a doctoral program must also ask itself what the possibilities are of the school being able to compete for extramural funds for research. The largest source of such funds is the National Institutes of Health, and competition for funding becomes more intense each year. The largest share of NIH dollars, including those disbursed by the National Center for Nursing Research, goes to a few nationally prominent research-intensive universities. This reality should not discourage a school from attempting to enter this competition, however, a realistic appraisal of a school's chances to compete successfully in this quest for research dollars should be considered in planning for the new program.

Faculty

The quality of faculty, specifically the graduate faculty, is the single most important factor to be considered in mounting a doctoral program. There should be a sufficient number of faculty representing a variety of subspecialty areas in nursing, as well as a few faculty holding a doctorate in allied disciplines such as physiology, sociology, or psychology. The mix of faculty can be crucial in the overall picture. Larger schools will generally have a broader mix of faculty although one or two subspecialty areas may predominate.

The eventual admission of students would ideally be matched to the resources faculty represent. That is, it would be appropriate to recruit students who wish to have a cognate minor in gerontology when there is faculty strength in this area. It would be inappropriate, on the other hand, to admit students wishing to concentrate in perinatal nursing when there are few or no faculty who are active researchers/clinicians in this field. Assessment of faculty resources including the long-range outlook for composition of the faculty is indicated. While composition of the faculty at the time the program will admit students is important, it need not overweigh the near-range outlook. If an articulated strategy for building certain areas of competence within the faculty is in place, planning to offer specific areas of concentration adjunct to the nursing core is justified.

Contingencies. Planning for contingencies enters into each phase of the assessment for readiness. With respect to faculty, there is no guarantee as to which faculty will remain for an extended time and which will seek opportunities elsewhere. Again, historical data can be helpful. If there has been relatively little faculty turnover in recent years, and there is a sizable cohort of tenured faculty who are research productive, one can assume that this trend will continue. Of equal importance, and an incentive to continue to plan for initiating the doctoral program, is a trend indicating a steady rate of hiring younger, doctorally qualified faculty from a wide geographic area. Such a trend indicates the drawing power of the school/university. It also fosters greater intellectual diversity and the infusion of fresh ideas into curriculum.

The number of nursing faculty having appointments in the graduate school should be considered, as well as the number of faculty who are likely to secure such status within the near future. Requirements for graduate faculty status vary among institutions. In some universities it is a status almost guaranteed a faculty member if he or she possesses a doctoral degree and has had several years of graduate level teaching. In other schools, the criteria for appointment may be fairly stringent and the status not easily acquired. Whatever the criteria for appointment, such a position is a generally recognized symbol of academic achievement. In some graduate schools, the requirement exists that only those with graduate faculty status may chair dissertation committees. Thus, in universities where this requirement exists it can profoundly affect monitoring and progression of doctoral students in nursing. Even though nursing has been accepted in the university relatively recently as a professional discipline, its faculty must meet the same criteria for appointment, promotion, and tenure as faculty in all other disciplines (Conway & Andruskiw, 1983).

Physical Facilities

The adequacy of physical facilities and their adjuncts to support both faculty and students in their research endeavors must be addressed. (It is assumed that classrooms and other basic equipment supporting the instructional mission of the university are adequate.)

Availability and *access* are two separate and equally important concerns. In a research-intensive university there may be extensive laboratory space yet most if not all of that space may already be dedicated to specific departments and kinds of research. Such space is not readily expandable, nor can the dean or faculty of the school of nursing expect to get space allocated even though their need for such space is justifiable. Space projections are usually based upon the thrust of the research to be undertaken by doctoral students—as well as that of faculty. For example, if physiological research is to be a major focus, bench laboratory space and equipment will be required; if behavioral research is to be a major focus, other kinds of space will be needed. Such space can vary from interviewing rooms to sleep laboratories.

The equipment and materials that will be required by students can be expensive. Funds for these must be considered a cost of the program. In those instances where the doctoral student will be working closely with a faculty whose research is funded, the cost consideration may be less formidable. Doctoral students universally need access to a sophisticated computer network. (This access should be without charge to the student.) In addition, students should have the assistance of a data programmer or analyst. This, too, should be available without a charge to the student, or, if a fee is to be levied it should be included as a fee along with tuition.

The library—the extent and quality of its holdings—is a critical adjunct to any doctoral program. Faculty responsible for the program of study should take an inventory of the library's holdings and compose a list of additional books and/or serials that should be available. The larger libraries should make study carrels available to doctoral students; if such space is in short supply, it may be found elsewhere on the campus. The storage and safekeeping of data printouts, especially during the dissertation stage, is a vital consideration as well.

Increasingly schools of nursing are establishing autonomous centers (or offices) for research and staffing them with faculty and other personnel with specific expertise in such areas as research design, statistics, and computer data analysis. Access to experts in such a center should be made available to doctoral students. In many instances the center itself can benefit from the involvement of doctoral students as research assistants. Advanced students frequently can assist master's students in their thesis work. The center can be expected to have a small library, microcomputers, a conference room, and one or more clerical staff. Again, the scope of services and staffing of a center depend largely upon school size and its dollar resources. (Where costs associated with all of the above may be considerable, the dean may need two or three years lead time to plan budgetary allocations and reallocations in advance of student enrollment.)

ELEMENTS OF A PLAN

At the point in the stage of deliberations about the feasibility of initiating a doctoral program when a decision has been made to commit to the task of getting ready, a step by step plan is desirable—in fact, a *must*. There can be several approaches to preparing such a plan. The dean, or other official, may delegate the responsibility of developing the plan to an associate or assistant dean. Or, the dean may constitute a task force of faculty with one or more administrative resource persons to develop the plan. In general, the latter approach is likely to be more productive. Faculty commitment and involvement early in the planning stage more likely results in a sound plan and a technically strong proposal.

Essential elements of a plan include at least the following:

1. An outline of the steps that must be accomplished up to and including presentation of the proposal to the university and/or system's officials for approval

2. Setting target dates for accomplishment of each step

3. Development of a sound written rationale for the program

4. Summarization of feasibility data—or collection of data if it has not been done

5. Development of assessment model consisting of criteria for assessing readiness within the school/university

6. Assignment of specific tasks to members of the task force, as well as other selected individuals as appropriate

7. Determination of the content and timing of periodic reports to all faculty

8. Identification of individuals and groups to whom formal presentations must be made prior to presenting the proposal to the authorizing officials

9. Drafting the entire proposal, including curriculum developed, to the extent required by the university

10. Compilation of a list of faculty qualified to teach doctoral students, including their research in progress, publications, and areas of specialization

11. Identification of a consultant who will be asked to critique both readiness factors and the written proposal, allowing time for revisions in the proposal following consultant's appraisal

The scope of the plan as outlined above is extensive enough to require the full time assignment of a faculty member to direct and coordinate the efforts of all individuals involved. In addition, a large amount of secretarial assistance will be required to produce drafts of materials.

Concurrent with the planning process carried out by the task force, the dean and the financial officer have the task of outlining fiscal resources that will be needed. Generally speaking, a three or four year timetable should be outlined in which additional faculty and other needed resources are identified, together with the amount of additional funds that will be required in each year. The fiscal plan should also indicate in which quarters or years existing funds will be reallocated. Contingent plans should be outlined as well. For example, if the operating budget should be less than anticipated in any given year, alternatives to the original plan should be specified.

ROLE FOR CONSULTANT

A consultant external to the university can be extremely useful in the assessment process. The consultant retained by the school should be a nurse educator who is experienced in doctoral education in nursing and, preferably, an educator who directs such a program.

The extent of the consultant's expected duties will determine the point in the timetable at which the consultant will be asked to make a site visit, or, review materials. For example, if the consultant's critique of the assessment-for-readiness model is desired, the model can be sent to him or her for review before data collection is begun. On the other hand, if only a final review of the proposal or the curriculum is desired, then the consultant's services will be contracted for a later date in the process.

The decision whether a site visit is needed is, of course, a discretionary one left to the dean and faculty. The attendance of an outside expert (i.e., the consultant) at one or more presentations of the proposal to groups in the university may lend additional credibility to the faculty's plan. The presence of the consultant can also encourage discussion of issues on which there may be divergent opinions among faculty in other disciplines. One example of such an issue might be the question of whether every student should be expected to have a minor external to nursing. Another might be the nature of the requirement for a supervised research experience for students prior to the dissertation. The latter question is one that frequently leads to much discussion particularly where bench scientists serve on graduate curriculum committees. One reason for such discussion is that predoctoral research training of a candidate in one of the basic sciences differs markedly from research training for the predoctoral nurse candidate. The norm for training in a basic science such as physiology, for example, is a one-on-one experience —mentor and trainee in the laboratory.

The final determination of when the consultant should be involved and how much time will be expected of him or her will depend upon the specific services desired. These expectations will be mutually agreed upon by the consultant and dean prior to a formal agreement or contract.

SUMMARY

While it is a fairly simple task to outline the general nature of the setting and the resources that are necessary to mount a quality doctoral program in nursing, there are some intangibles that can be identified but not quantified. Of these intangibles the *ethos* that is readily perceptible on a given campus can be a harbinger of success—or failure—of a new program. On some campuses there is a palpable sense of community embracing faculty, administration, and students. Distinguishing features of these high-morale environments are strong leadership combined with a "flat" organizational structure. Hierarchical distinctions are largely absent and no one person or group dominates (Rice & Austin, 1988). A sense of unified purpose is the glue that appears to hold the community together.

This energizing *ethos* is not something that can be readily constructed from a formula or prescription. But in those universities where it is found, it bodes well for a new program. Conversely, where students, faculty, and staff perceive themselves in competition for professional esteem and scarce dollars, the learning environment will be less enhancing.

Assessment of readiness to start a doctoral program, or any academic program for that matter, requires thoughtful consideration of a variety of factors. Although a school of nursing may very much want to become part of the mainstream of doctorate granting schools, ambition must be tempered with reality. The realities for each school and university will differ. Integrity of product demands that deans, administrators, and faculty conduct a careful appraisal of the resources presently available to them as well as to those that must be made available over the long run. Both the science and the discipline of nursing will be poorly served unless quality of program is to be the major goal.

REFERENCES

Baldridge, J. V., Curtis, D., Ecker, G., & Riley, G. (1978). *Policy making and effective leadership.* San Francisco: Jossey-Bass.

Carnegie Foundation for the Advancement of Teaching. (1975). *More than survival.* San Francisco: Jossey-Bass.

Conway, M., & Andruskiw, O. (1983). *Administrative theory and practice: Issues in higher education in nursing.* New York: Appleton, Century, Crofts.

Council of Graduate Schools in the United States. (1977). *A policy statement.* Washington, DC: Author.

Mayhew, L. B., & Ford, P. J. (1974). *Reform in graduate and professional education.* San Francisco: Jossey-Bass.

Mingle, J. R., & Associates. (1981). *Challenges of retrenchment.* San Francisco: Jossey-Bass.

Mingle, J. R., & Norris, D. M. (1981). Institutional strategies for responding to decline. In J. R. Mingle & Associates (Eds.), *Challenges of retrenchment.* San Francisco: Jossey-Bass.

National League for Nursing. (1988). *Nursing student census with policy implications.* New York: National League for Nursing, Division of Research.

Rice, E. R., & Austin, A. E. (1988). High faculty morale: What exemplary colleges do right. *Change, 20,* 51–58.

U.S. Department of Health and Human Services. (July, 1988). *Secretary's Commission on Nursing, Interim Report.* Washington, DC: Author.

U.S. Institute of Medicine, Division of Health Care Services. (1983). Washington, DC: National Academy Press.

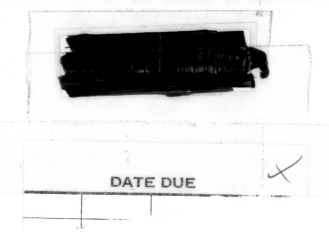

DATE DUE